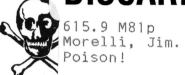

Poison!

HOW TO HANDLE THE HAZARDOUS SUBSTANCES IN YOUR HOME

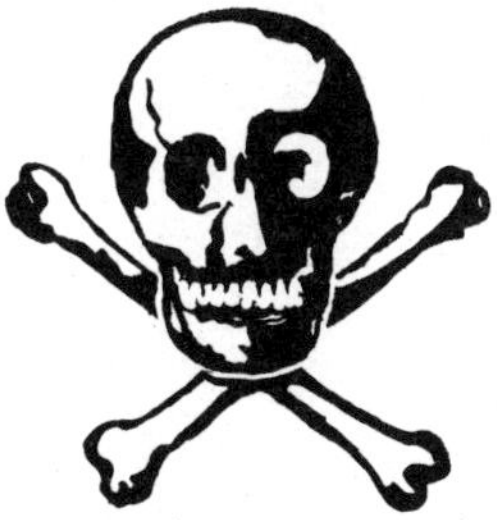

Jim Morelli

ANDREWS AND McMEEL
A Universal Press Syndicate Company
Kansas City

 For information, write Andrews and McMeel, a Universal Press Syndicate Company, 4520 Main Street, Kansas City, Missouri 64111.

Library of Congress Cataloging-in-Publication Data

Morelli, Jim.

Poison! : how to handle the hazardous substances in your home / Jim Morelli

p. cm.

Includes bibliographical references and index.

ISBN: 0-8362-2721-2 (pbk.)

1. Toxicology—Popular works. 2. Household supplies—Toxicology—Popular works. 3. Housing and health—Popular works. I. Title.

RA1213.M67 1997

615.9—dc20 96-44337

CIP

First Printing, April 1997

Second Printing, May 1997

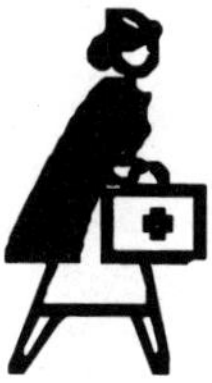

For Linda,

the antidote

for all that ails me.

Love ya, Scooter.

Contents

THIS BOOK IS NOT MEANT AS A SUBSTITUTE FOR COMPETENT MEDICAL CARE. ALL POISONINGS SHOULD BE HANDLED IN CONJUNCTION WITH A POISON CONTROL CENTER OR A MEDICAL PROFESSIONAL.

Acknowledgments

Special thanks to Duckby, copy editor number one, who has suffered through numerous projects on my behalf and fed me cake and frozen yogurt along the way. Thanks also to Jill Hannity, my news editor in Atlanta, for always giving me the time to pursue outside projects, and to Rick Hill at Andrews and McMeel for giving me *this* outside project—and treating it with enthusiasm and care. Thanks to Julie Vaillancourt of Washington, D.C., for turning me on to poison control way back when. Thanks also to the Mercer University Library and its staff for their assistance with this project, and the National Capital Poison Center in Washington, D.C., for happily answering my questions.

I'm one of those lucky people who has a great family, and for that I am grateful. Thanks to Lorraine and Stephen Morelli, my mother and father; brothers Bob, Tom, and Jeff; sister Chris; nieces Lissy and Gabby; and my nephew, Sam. Thanks also to Clay Parker, a loyal friend, who tolerated my spotty record at returning phone calls while I was immersed in this project.

Working in a poison control center can be a phone-slamming kind of job, and I am fortunate to have shared the experience with some great people over the years. They are: Diane Bartell, Bill Partridge, Gary Brown, Dusti Owens, Denise Martin, Kim Vanderburgh, Gerry Buller, Johnetta Miller, Julia Heard, Rob Turner, Joan Carter, Amy Steinkellner, J. T. Palmer, Gary Bumgarner, Roselyn Liew-Pardue, and the King of the toxic jungle himself, Robert H. Baker.

J.M.
August 1996
Atlanta

Introduction

Gum! Forbidden gum! How lucky I was to have found a box of gum. *Gum!* What in heck were we doing with gum in the house? Who cared? Not me. All I knew was *I* had found it—not my brothers or sister but *me.* It was mine. Knowing I'd have to share it with my siblings if they found out the gum existed, I crawled behind a living room chair and ate the entire box.

The gum was an unusual flavor called Feen-a-Mint.

I emerged from that rather stormy introduction to the world of laxatives with a deep-seated fear of poisons. And overall, it's a fear that has served me well. During adolescence, this fear kept me from going along with the crowd when, for example, the gang popped Placidyl, a powerful sleeping pill, before going out for a drive in the snow.

But sooner or later, you have to find a rational way to deal with your fears, and I think, subconsciously, that's why I started working in poison control. To paraphrase former senator Howard Baker, I needed to find out what it was I had to fear and when I had to fear it.

Now I know, and I'm sharing it with you. That's really the purpose of this book: to add a note of rationality to the mysterious world of poisons by tearing down some enduring myths. In these pages you'll learn that a swallow of bleach is no big deal, that munching on a poinsettia leaf won't kill you, and, conversely, why it's important never to eat a piece of fish that smells like pepper.

Because when it comes to poisons, knowledge is the best antidote to fear. But heck, if you prefer fear as a motivator, there's this gum. . . .

A Treatment Primer: Essential Facts

When to Induce Vomiting

Check your medicine cabinet. Got a bottle of ipecac syrup? Ipecac, a chemical derived from a plant, causes vomiting. We use it in treating some home poisonings to get toxic materials out of the stomach. Note I said *some* home poisonings, not *all*. In fact, there are times when using ipecac syrup is downright dangerous. When someone is at risk of having a seizure, for example, or is drowsy, the last thing you want is to have them vomiting as well. So the first rule for using ipecac: Never give ipecac syrup without consulting a poison center first.

The second rule: Follow dosing instructions to the letter. Most children usually vomit after a single one-tablespoonful dose of ipecac. But it isn't ipecac alone that stimulates vomiting, you need fluid too, preferably four to eight ounces of water or juice. (There's some argument as to whether milk delays ipecac's action, so stick with clear liquids.)

Vomiting will usually occur within half an hour. Once it starts, encourage—don't force—sips of water between each bout of vomiting. This insures a total cleanout and helps you gauge the end point of ipecac's action: When nothing but water comes up, you know the stomach's empty. *If it looks like the child can't handle sips of fluid while vomiting, don't push it.* Vomiting is uncomfortable—and potentially dangerous—enough without forcing fluid back down the throat.

This takes us to rule three: Keep the stomach empty for a total of two hours *after* you give the ipecac. Ipecac's irritant effect on the stomach lingers for that long, meaning that anything ingested during that time will come right back up. After two hours, test the stomach with a bit of fluid. If it stays down, you're all set. If not, wait another fifteen minutes and try again.

Rule four: Supervise sleep. Ipecac—and the stress of vomiting itself—makes children tired. It's okay to let them sleep, but: *don't leave them alone* and *never let them sleep on their backs.* Any residual fluid in the stomach could be vomited up during sleep and might cause choking.

Okay, you've given the ipecac, waited half an hour, and nothing has happened. What's wrong? The three biggest reasons ipecac won't work are:

1. Too little ipecac was given. Remember, one *table*spoonful is needed for most children; smaller amounts for infants (and only under the instruction of a poison center).

2. Not enough fluid was given. This is probably the biggest reason ipecac doesn't work. Remember, 4 to 8 ounces of clear fluid is needed for a good "return." If a child absolutely refuses to take any fluid following a dose of ipecac, go to the emergency room and have them handle the poisoning there.

3. The ipecac was out of date. If it's old, it won't work.

Occasionally, you might do everything right and the child *still* won't vomit. In those cases, it's acceptable to give another tablespoonful of ipecac, followed by another glass of fluid. But check with your poison center first. And keep in mind that redosing with ipecac sensitizes the stomach for even longer. Three or four hours may pass before things settle down to the point where eating is possible.

And finally, one more rule: Ipecac is the *only* way you should ever induce vomiting. No raw eggs, no salt water, no clunky adult fingers shoved down a child's throat: *these are dangerous methods and should never be used.*

Now go out and get that ipecac if you don't have it.

Treating Eyes and Skin

Eye Rinsing

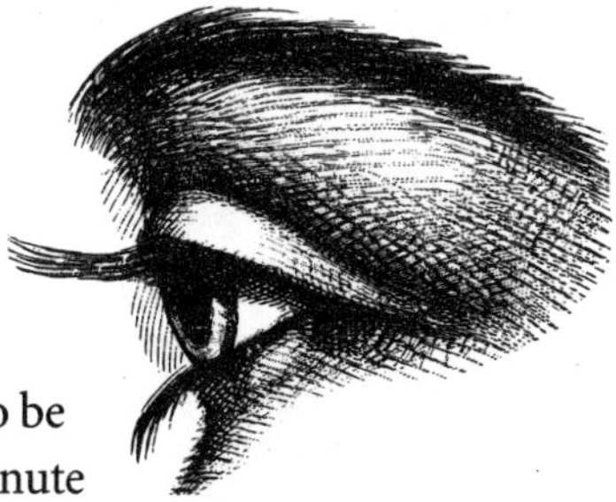

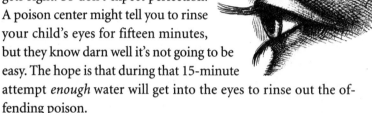

There's no such thing as a perfect eye rinse. Eye rinsing is a messy, disruptive procedure that almost nobody gets right. So don't expect perfection. A poison center might tell you to rinse your child's eyes for fifteen minutes, but they know darn well it's not going to be easy. The hope is that during that 15-minute attempt *enough* water will get into the eyes to rinse out the offending poison.

While there's no easy way to do an eye rinse, here are a few tips:

- Wrap the child up in a towel mummy-style. A package is always easier to handle than a bunch of flailing limbs.
- Use lukewarm water. It's close in temperature to tears.
- Pour the water from a glass onto the bridge of the nose, a little at a time, letting it dribble down into the eyes. This is a heck of a lot less intimidating than thrusting a child's head under the faucet.
- The more crying the better. Crying rinses the eyes.
- Older children might do better in the shower. Turn on a low-intensity lukewarm spray and encourage the child to look up at the water every so often. *Keep the shower spray gentle.* We don't want to damage the eyes.
- Never force open a child's eyelids. If there's absolutely no way you can do the eye rinse at home, let an emergency room do it or call 911.
- Eyedrops are *not* an eye rinse. The only way to "get the red out" after a toxic exposure is with water.

A Treatment Primer: Essential Facts

Treating Skin

This is simple. Thorough soap and water *washing* of the skin means just that—but do it gently. *Irrigating* the skin means passing a continuous stream of water over it.

Hospital Remedies for Poisoning

The Stomach Pump

The sanitized term for pumping out the stomach is "gastric lavage." Think of it as a belly enema: A tube is forced down the throat and into the stomach; then a washing solution is pushed through. The goal is to rinse the inside of the stomach clean before sucking the whole mess—solution and stomach contents—back out.

Activated Charcoal

Activated charcoal is arguably the most important weapon in a hospital's arsenal against poisons. Activated charcoal adsorbs poisons. In fact, there are very few poisons that *won't* stick to activated charcoal. So almost every time gastric lavage is performed, it's followed up by a dose of activated charcoal. In small children, it's given through a tube; older children and adults can drink it on their own.

Activated charcoal comes ready packaged in a laxative solution with sorbitol. Sorbitol's the same sweetening agent you'll find in many "sugar-free" gums and candies (so don't eat too many of those!). Sorbitol's an important ingredient in activated charcoal therapy because the goal is not just to adsorb the poison but to get the whole package—charcoal and toxin—out of the body as quickly as possible.

Part 1

Around the House

1

Animals

When it comes to poisonous animals, the United States gets off easy. With just a few native poisonous snakes, spiders, and scorpions, fatalities from animal bites and stings are rare. Not so in other countries. In India, for example, cobra bites and scorpion stings are a serious problem. In Australia, the deadly sea wasp, a type of jellyfish, delivers a poison so potent it can kill a swimmer in less than an hour. Also in Australia lives one of the world's most toxic spiders, the funnel web, a big lumbering beast that attaches itself so firmly to the skin that it sometimes has to be torn off. So next time you stumble across a fire ant nest or a brown recluse spider, keep things in perspective: When it comes to poisonous animals, we're lucky.

Insect and Spider Bites

Bees and Wasps

Bees and wasps kill more people in the United States each year than any other animal. When you get right down to it, they're all killer bees. It isn't that their venom is so strong, it's that it affects some people so strongly. By and large, these deaths occur from allergic reactions.

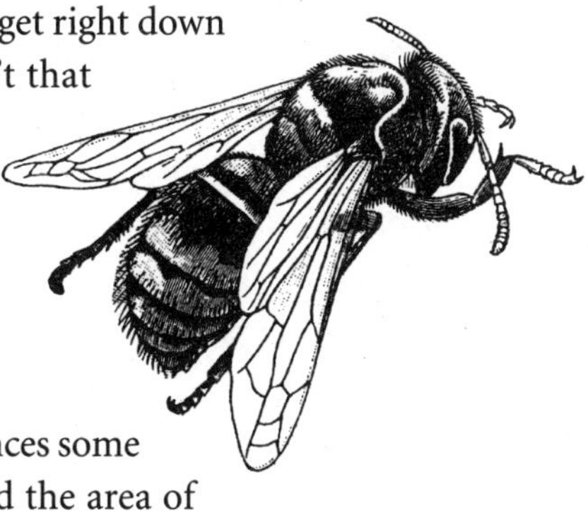

Treatment for Allergic Victims

Anyone stung by a bee experiences some degree of swelling, mainly around the area of the sting. But those who are allergic develop massive, widespread swelling that may involve the throat. It becomes difficult to swallow or breathe, and the blood pressure may fall so rapidly that it causes shock. A bee sting in an allergic individual is a medical emergency. Waste no time. Call 911.

What about a home bee-sting kit? Go for it. These injections of adrenaline can save lives if used properly. However, you still need to dial 911 and get your bee-sting victim to a hospital. And learn to use the kit *before* an emergency strikes.

Treatment for the Rest of Us

For some reason, bee stings bring out the creative folk doctor in people. Everybody, it seems, has a novel way of treating them. In the South, some believe in the pain-relieving properties of wet tobacco; others prefer a good long soak in bleach. Do yourself a favor: Avoid these folk remedies. They can actually make the situation worse by irritating and possibly infecting the sting.

Instead, wash the sting area thoroughly with soap and water. Try to remove the stinger (if one has been left behind), using a pair of clean tweezers. If you can't easily remove it, let a doctor or nurse handle the chore. Disinfect the area with rubbing alcohol or hydrogen peroxide to help prevent an infection. And finally, to relieve pain, make a paste of water and powdered meat tenderizer, and slather it over the sting. Bee venom is made up of proteins, and meat tenderizers break proteins down.

See a doctor if one of the following is true:

- You've swallowed the insect and it has stung you in the mouth or throat. The resultant swelling can make breathing and swallowing difficult.
- The sting is in a vulnerable spot: near the eyes, for example, or the genitals.
- Hours later, the sting isn't getting any better. It's warm, swollen, and painful to the touch. It might be infected.

It's a Fact

• Bees live in an amazingly well-ordered society. There's the queen; there are the male drones, whose sole purpose in life is to inseminate the queen in a rapturous ceremony and then die; and finally there are the worker bees, the ones you see dipping into flowers. The worker bees are all females, and they're the only ones that can sting.

• How's this for genetic engineering? A colony of bees actually creates a queen by feeding a female larva a steady diet of royal jelly, a hormone-rich paste secreted from glands in the worker bees' mouths. The other female larvae subsist largely on an inferior diet of nectar. They will become the worker bees.

• The "honey belt" stretches from the Canadian provinces of Alberta, Saskatchewan, and Manitoba down to Minnesota and the Dakotas. More honey is produced in this region than any other place in North America.

• Yes, it's true; honey is, in a sense, bee vomit. It's manufactured in a special "honey stomach" from nectar gathered by worker bees. After the nectar is broken down into simple sugars, it's regurgitated into the cells of the honeycomb. Eventually, as water evaporates, it becomes honey.

• Bees are, perhaps, the single most important insect in the world. The reason: pollination. Many plant species depend on bees for their survival.

• The main difference between a bee and a wasp: Bees are sugar-freak vegetarians who subsist on nectar and pollen; wasps are carnivores who dine on other insects.

• You've disturbed a nest of bees or wasps and they've come out fighting, stinging you multiple times. It's hard to say exactly how many stings will kill an otherwise healthy person, but it might be a good idea to head to an emergency room with, say, ten or more stings.

- You've never been stung before but there's a family history of bee allergies. Even if you're in no distress, go to the emergency room and sit in the waiting area for a few hours. That way, if you start experiencing problems you can receive prompt attention.
- You've developed major swelling from a sting, defined as puffiness that creeps past the major joint nearest the sting. If you've been stung on the foot and your calf is swollen, for example, you probably need to see a doctor.

What about those killer bees? They're here! Since 1957, when they were first accidentally released into Brazil, the African honeybee, better known as the killer bee, has been edging its way northward. The ferocious critters recently crossed the Rio Grande, and bee attacks in Texas have been reported.

Picture a bee on PCP and you have a good idea why these insects are called killers: They are aggressive, tenacious, and difficult to control once riled up. Worse, they drive out other, more productive honeybees. So in Texas or other states in the Southwest be careful around bees. As for the rest of America: Stay tuned—the killer bees are inching north.

Black Widow Spider (Latrodectus mactans)

You're out camping and you have to use the bathroom, so you head off to the nearest privy. It's dark inside and you can't see the spider lolling upside down in the toilet hole. It's black, shiny as a lump of coal, and has a dash of red across its belly. You sit down, never realizing you're about to become its next victim.

Treatment

Getting bitten by a black widow spider is a heck of a way to end a camping trip. Within two hours, painful spasms grip the chest, back, and abdomen. You feel like you're going to die. Are you? The answer, in all probability, is no. Within 24 hours or so, the painful

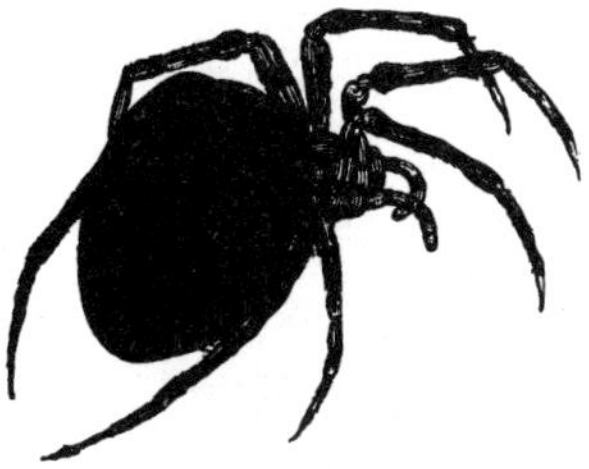

symptoms will subside. But the intense pain and attendant anxiety associated with a black widow spider bite calls for immediate medical attention. Take anyone bitten by a black widow spider to the emergency room.

Treatment in the hospital includes use of muscle relaxants like methocarbamol (Robaxin) and diazepam (Valium), as well as painkillers. If these things don't ease the pain, there's an antivenin available, but it's usually reserved only for the very young, very old, or very sick.

Avoiding black widows is easy. Black widows, like other spiders, have developed an undeserved reputation for viciousness. In fact, they are shy creatures that just happen to pack a hell of a punch. The attitude of the black widow spider is simple: You don't bother me, I don't bother you. So don't get anywhere near a black widow's web. If you touch it, the spider may think you're a captured fly and scurry over for a snap.

If you live anywhere in the continental United States, you've got black widow spiders living nearby. But most of the time they stay out of sight, under woodpiles, rubbish, old logs, and, as we learned from the unfortunate camper, in the toilet holes of outhouses. In fact, black widow spider bites occurred more frequently before the days of indoor plumbing.

Spotting one can sometimes be difficult. By and large, a black widow spider will look like a black widow spider: a jet-black shiny spider about an inch in diameter that sports on its

It's a Fact

• Female black widows—the ones with the poisonous bite—can live for up to three years. The males, as you might have guessed from the species' name, have far shorter life spans. In fact, the female usually kills the male shortly after mating.

• Black widow spiders rarely leave their webs.

• Baby black widow spiders are usually not black but have red and white stripes.

underside an hourglass-shaped marking the color of blood. But not always. Sometimes the marking can be orange or yellow and will look more like a series of lines or dots. Sometimes the whole spider will be red or orange. In this case, you've got, technically, a red-legged widow spider—just as poisonous, but usually found only in the southern states. A less-poisonous relative is the gray widow spider. The best advice on identifying any of these widows: Look for a globous back end. It's far more pronounced than on other spiders.

And about that venom. Black widow spider venom blocks nerve transmission, hence the painful muscle spasms. Occasionally, a black widow spider may bite but not inject enough venom to cause a reaction. But play it safe. If you're bitten, head to the emergency room. If no reaction occurs within two hours, you're probably home free.

Brown Recluse Spider (Loxosceles reclusa)

Ah, winter. Time to hit the attic and haul out those winter coats, hats, gloves, and blankets. A word of advice before you put any of these articles near your body: Take them outside and shake them out. Otherwise, you might find yourself sharing your bed with a brown recluse spider. That's especially true if you live in the heavily infested belt, a swath of southern and midwestern states that includes Arkansas, Tennessee, Missouri, Mississippi, Kansas, Oklahoma, Louisiana, Alabama, and Georgia.

Actually, it's hard to find a state that *doesn't* have a brown recluse population; this spider is one of the great hitchhikers of the animal kingdom. It likes to hide in boxes, old clothes, and furniture and is thus easily transported to far-flung and even ridiculously cold destinations. Brown recluse spiders have been found in Bangor, Maine, for example. And a spate of bites in Connecticut was traced to lumber transported up from Georgia.

Outdoors, your best protection against a spider bite is gloves. Brown recluses hide in some pretty strange places, like gutters and between walls. So always wear gloves when reaching into a dark, undisturbed place.

One of the most stubborn myths regarding the brown recluse is that its venom "eats" flesh away. It's an understandable misconception, given that these bite wounds resemble ulcers. But the venom doesn't so much eat away at flesh as starve it to death by cutting off blood and oxygen. Complicating the situation is the body's natural reaction. Once it realizes it's been poisoned, the body sends in defensive troops called polymorphonuclear leukocytes (PMNs for short). These cells attack the wound area with chemicals designed to improve healing. Only problem is, these cells wind up doing just the opposite: scarring the battlefield with chemicals that only add to the swelling.

Treatment

The first rule is: Don't panic. A few years back, a report came out that a California woman bitten by a brown recluse spider ended up with "bilateral limb loss," an antiseptic way of saying she lost her arms and legs. But actually, brown recluse bites rarely cause serious problems. Only about 10 percent of cases will need continuing medical treatment, and even fewer will suffer skin loss so severe as to require grafting. So if you've been bitten by a brown recluse, don't panic. The odds are with you on this one. Instead, take the following measures.

1. Chill the wound by applying an ice pack on an intermittent basis. The goal here is not to freeze the tissue but to cool it down. This may help restrict the flow of brown recluse venom from the bite site. Important: *Don't leave ice on the wound for very long.* The last thing you need on top of a brown recluse wound is frostbite.

2. Get to a doctor, if you're certain it's a brown recluse that bit you. Those who suffer most severely from brown recluse bites are the ones who don't get early treatment. If you're not sure it was a brown recluse, it's probably all right to wait for, say, ten to fifteen

hours to see what develops. Use ice as instructed and take analgesics like ibuprofen, aspirin, or acetaminophen. Warning: *If you develop a rash on your body or symptoms that mimic the flu shortly after a bite, see a doctor.* About 20 percent of brown recluse victims develop a "serum sickness" to the venom. It's usually mild and normally resolves within a day or two.

3. After ten to fifteen hours, if you still feel fine, carefully examine the bite. If it looks like a bruise is developing in the center, you may have a brown recluse bite. The dark-colored center indicates an area of tissue that is already dead. Red and white rings radiating outward indicate the body is in full panic over this toxic invader and the result is intense inflammation, warmth, and pain. The simple rule: *If the bite has turned into something that looks like a bull's-eye, head to the doctor.*

But keep in mind: The brown recluse spider has stumped the medical profession. As a result, many brown recluse victims are treated with ineffectual drugs while the wound continues to fester. If your doctor automatically concludes you need an antibiotic for the brown recluse bite, share this little nugget of information: Brown recluse venom is so powerful that it kills most bacteria. So, while using an antibiotic will help prevent a major infection on the open wound, *an antibiotic will do nothing to stop brown recluse venom from destroying tissue.*

Instead, ask your doctor to look into the use of dapsone. Ever heard of Hansen's disease? That's the official name for leprosy. Dapsone, a drug used to treat Hansen's disease, appears to have some beneficial effects on brown recluse bites by inhibiting the migration of those PMNs to the bite area. That reduces inflammation and gives the wound a chance to heal. One drawback to dapsone: It can cause destruction of red blood cells as a side effect. But so can brown recluse venom.

4. Beyond dapsone and other drugs, there's hyperbaric oxygen. What do deep-sea divers with the bends and brown recluse bite victims have in common? They both benefit from spending time

It's a Fact

• The brown recluse is also called the fiddleback spider, because of the violin-shaped marking on its back, just behind its eyes. (Not that you'll get close enough to see those eyes, but, unlike other spiders, the brown recluse has six pairs instead of eight.)

• The brown recluse probably migrated to the United States in the 1920s, perhaps on a fruit boat from South America. It may have landed first in New Orleans or Biloxi, then made its way north on barges floating up the Mississippi River.

• A relation, *Tegenaria agrestis,* or the hobo spider, primarly lives in the Pacific Northwest. Like the brown recluse, it causes ulcerating wounds. However, its bites are considered less severe.

• The brown recluse spider is a wanderer. It leaves its ground-level web to search for prey, usually at night.

• Deaths rarely occur with brown recluse bites, but the venom has been associated with a rare but potentially deadly condition called disseminated intravascular coagulation, or DIC. Translation: lots of blood clots.

• Most brown recluse bites occur in the fall and spring, due, most probably, to that stored-clothing thing.

in a hyperbaric oxygen chamber. In the case of brown recluse bites, there's a nearly 100 percent cure rate. So why isn't everyone with a spider bite jammed into a hyperbaric tube? Because there aren't enough of them to go around, and most brown recluse bites can be treated in less drastic ways. But for those with persistent bites, or those unlucky enough to have been bitten on the face, genitals, or another sensitive spot, hyperbaric oxygen is the way to go. Here's how it works. Inside the hyperbaric chamber, oxygen is forced into the tissues under pressure. This helps break down some of the chemical bonds in brown recluse venom and, by supplying oxygen to the damaged tissues, allows healing to occur. Consider asking about hyperbaric oxygen if your wound isn't healing.

Above all else, be your own doctor. That is, be an active participant in your care. Ask questions and make recommendations to your doctor if it doesn't look like the wound is getting any better. Remember, as the weeks go by and you keep swallowing those putrid-smelling cephalexin capsules (a favorite antibiotic "treatment" for brown recluse bites), the spider's venom is sinking deeper and deeper into the tissues, causing more damage along the way. So be suspicious of your care if weeks go by and the wound isn't getting any better.

Tarantula Spider (Eurypelma californicum)

There must be some misunderstanding. It seems to be the tarantula's mission in life to take all the hits for the spider world. The big hairy fellow is the dubious star of everything from *Arachnophobia* to that *Brady Bunch* Hawaii episode in which Peter wakes to find a tarantula crawling on his chest.

Actually, you could do much worse than have a tarantula crawl across your pajamas. It's a rather gentle spider, actually, so much so that some people keep tarantulas as pets. Tarantula venom is weak. It will cause some pain, and the spider's hairs are irritating to the skin. But usually, bites from a tarantula are no worse than those from a bee.

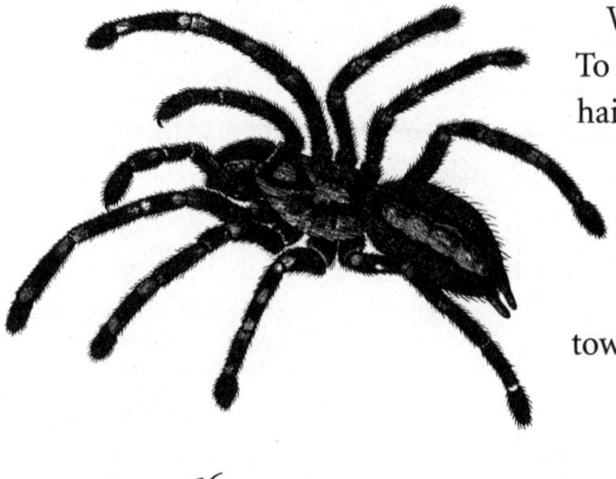

What, exactly, is a tarantula? To Americans, a tarantula is a hairy reddish-black spider that lives in the desert. To Europeans, the tarantula is actually a form of wolf spider that got its name from the town of Taranto, Italy. The European tarantula was thought to be so poisonous that bite victims went into a frenzied dance before collapsing. This belief in "tarantism" led to the popular Italian dance La Tarantella, in which participants literally dance until they drop. Only nobody really dies from the bite of a "taranto" spider. Like the tarantula, the Italian wolf spider's bite is about as bad as a bee's.

In the southern United States, some wolf spiders grow to be as big as tarantulas. And actually, they are more poisonous than the real tarantulas, causing wounds similar to that of a brown recluse. However, the body can detoxify wolf spider venom more easily than that of the recluse, so bites tend to heal quickly.

It's a Fact

- Few small creatures live as long as the tarantula. Some specimens have survived for thirty years.
- Tarantulas in South America grow as big as dinner plates. They feed on small rodents and birds.
- Tarantulas don't spin webs, per se. Instead, they live in underground burrows. At night, they come out and hunt for lizards, frogs, toads, insects, and small rodents.

Treatment

If you're bitten by a true tarantula, use basic first aid. Wash the wound with soap and water and apply a disinfectant like alcohol or hydrogen peroxide. For continued irritation, rub in some hydrocortisone cream and take an analgesic. The pain from a tarantula bite usually subsides within a few hours. If swelling, pain, and warmth linger longer than that, see a doctor. It might be infected.

Scorpions

What looks like a lobster and stings like a bee? You got it: scorpions. In the pantheon of creepy creatures, scorpions rank near the top. You might think you're safe from scorpions if you don't live in the desert, but you would be wrong. Scorpions thrive in

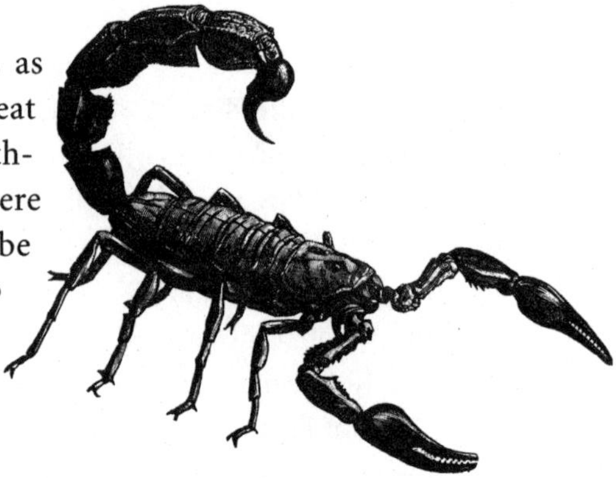

such temperate climates as British Columbia and Great Britain. Even in the southeastern United States, where winters can occasionally be harsh, scorpions turn up all over the place: in the kitchen, under the bed, inside closets, hanging on the ceiling.

Scorpions are ground dwellers and may enter homes by following plumbing pipes or openings in the foundation. New homes may be especially prone to an infestation; excavation work tends to dig up scorpions. While it's a little jarring to see a scorpion scurry across the kitchen floor, in most areas of the country they

It's a Fact

• Scorpions are among the oldest creatures on earth, with ancestors that go back 430 million years, and there's a good reason they've survived that long. Scorpions are virtually indestructible. They can survive freezing temperatures, heat that would kill other animals, and even a one- or two-day submersion in water.

• When newly hatched, scorpions stay on the backs of the mother in a large clump. But as adults, scorpions are loners.

• The largest scorpions are nearly a foot long and live in tropical Africa.

• Scorpion stings in India, South America, and other warm regions of the world are extremely dangerous. Also, when visiting Mexico, take special care to avoid scorpions, as some are more toxic than those found in the United States.

• *Centruroides* stings may be more severe in those with preexisting high blood pressure.

are harmless. They might sting you, but they're usually no more toxic than a bee.

The exception is in the desert Southwest, where the more toxic *Centruroides* genus of scorpion lives. *Centruroides* venom affects the heart, and death is possible (though rare) following a sting. Therefore, any scorpion sting that occurs in a *Centruroides*-infested area requires emergency room observation and treatment. Catch the scorpion if you can do so safely, so that it can be identified.

Treatment

Wash and disinfect the wound, using soap, water, and alcohol or hydrogen peroxide. Apply a paste made of baking soda and water. Pain from a scorpion sting normally dissipates within a few hours. If severe swelling, an extensive rash, or shortness of breath develops, head to the emergency room

Fire Ants

It's been almost sixty years since red fire ants first landed on U.S. soil. Since then, they've colonized more than one hundred million acres, mostly in the South. Southerners have learned to recognize and avoid the chief sign of a fire ant infestation: a mound of red dirt, sometimes piled a yard high.

The problem with fire ants is that they bite aggressively—and acrobatically. Envenomation takes place in two moves. First, the fire ant sinks its fangs (called mandibles) into the skin; then it swings around and injects venom. If you've ever been bitten by a fire ant, you know how it got its name. The venom causes immediate and fiery pain, swelling, and sometimes the formation of a pus-filled blister.

Fire ants themselves are not all that poisonous. However, deaths have occurred as the result of numerous stings. In Augusta, Georgia, for example, a murder case a few years back hinged around whether a man was pushed into a fire ant nest after a fight.

Back in the 1950s, when it seemed all things could be solved by science, Congress started a fire ant eradication program that by 1978 had cost $150 million. Take a careful walk in almost any open field in the South and you'll understand why one author has characterized that program as the Vietnam of pest control efforts. The fire ants, it seems, are here to stay.

Treatment

For large-scale stings, such as might occur from falling into a nest, it's best to get medical treatment at the emergency room. Most such victims will have no major problems, but toxic reactions are unpredictable, and a few hours of medical observation can't hurt.

Smaller exposures can be handled at home by a soak in the tub. Put something soothing in the water, like Aveeno or baking soda. After soaking, use over-the-counter anti-inflammatories like hydrocortisone cream or a topical anesthetic. For severe pain, take acetaminophen, aspirin, or ibuprofen. In general, pain from fire ant stings will resolve within an hour or two. As with any wound, watch for signs of infection: more pain, warmth, and redness. See a doctor if these develop.

Don't blame everything on the fire ant, though. Almost all ants are capable of stinging and biting. Some release formic acid into a bite, which can be counteracted with a baking-soda-and-water soak.

It's a Fact

• Red fire ants emigrated from South America and are believed to have entered the United States through the port of Mobile, Alabama.

• Wonder what's inside a fire ant nest? How about fifty thousand ants and three thousand queens.

• Cable companies hate fire ants, too. The creatures are attracted to electromagnetic fields, such as you might find around a buried phone line.

Saddleback Caterpillar (Sibine stimulea *larva*)

You've seen a monster while hiking in the Appalachian Mountains. He's green and has a big purple splotch on his back. Sticking out from either end of his body are hornlike protrusions.

That's not a monster, it's a saddleback caterpillar. And he won't hurt you unless you touch him. If you do, your hiking holiday will stall in fiery pain. Picture yourself igniting a matchbook and then applying the flaming object to the skin. That's what a saddleback sting feels like. Here's why: The saddleback is covered with hundreds of venom-containing hairs. When you brush against its body, these hairs detach into your skin.

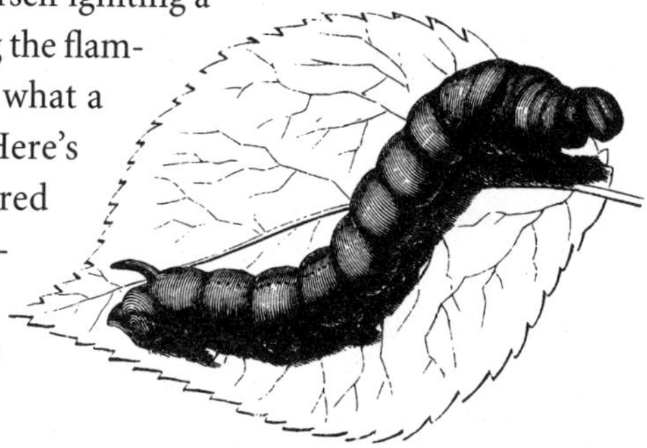

Treatment

The first thing to reach for after a saddleback caterpillar sting is first-aid tape—paper or plastic, it doesn't matter. Gently press a strip over the sting area, then lift it off slowly. The tape will remove any saddleback hairs that remain in the skin. Next, head to the nearest pharmacy, because a variety of nonprescription drugs will suffice as treatment for most caterpillar stings.

Start with an analgesic: acetaminophen, aspirin, ibuprofen, ketoprofen, or naproxen. These relieve pain and—aside from acetaminophen—inflammation as well.

Next, choose an antihistamine. Diphenhydramine (Benadryl) is a good choice; so is chlorpheniramine (Chlor-Trimeton). These products help reduce inflammation by countering the action of histamine, a chemical in the body that causes redness and swelling.

Add a topical steroid cream like hydrocortisone, and you should be well on the way to relief.

There is no antidote for saddleback caterpillar venom, nor is one generally needed. However, as with any insect bite or sting, some victims develop severe allergic reactions. If you notice swelling extending beyond the immediate sting area, a skin rash, or tightness in the chest, go immediately to the emergency room.

Warning: Never let the eyes come in contact with a saddleback caterpillar sting. The tiny hairs can damage the eyes. Anyone stung in or near the eyes should be treated in the emergency room.

Ticks

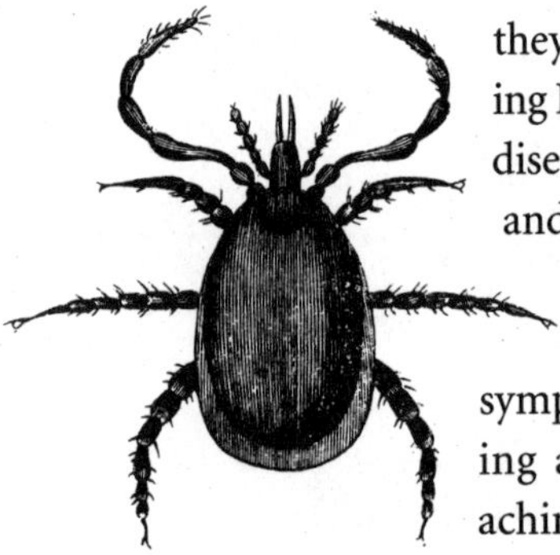

Ticks are not poisonous. The trouble is, they transmit several nasty diseases, including Rocky Mountain spotted fever and Lyme disease. Not all ticks transmit these diseases, and most tick bites *do not* result in illness, but you never can tell. Keep it in the back of your mind that if *any* unusual symptoms develop in the two weeks following a tick bite—especially fever, rash, or aching muscles, joints, or head—see a doctor. Meanwhile, you need to remove the creature, provided you can see it. Some ticks are so small—the deer tick, for example, which transmits Lyme disease—that it's nearly impossible to remove them without hurting the skin. See a doctor if that's the situation.

Treatment for Visible Ticks

Put away the matches. You are not going to burn the tick's butt in the hope it will back out of the skin. Just the opposite may happen; it may burrow deeper. Instead, using a pair of tweezers, gently but firmly pull the tick *straight out* from the skin. Your goal here is not to crush the creature, lest you spill more microorganisms into the wound.

Once the tick is out of the skin, wash and disinfect the bite area, using soap, water, and perhaps some rubbing alcohol or peroxide. If you think you can't remove the tick, leave it to a medical professional.

Prevention

It's simple: Wear more clothes. Long pants and long sleeves provide plenty of protection from ticks, and it's highly advisable in areas where Lyme disease is endemic—New England and the Middle Atlantic states especially—to cover yourself when in the woods.

Rabid Animals

The mad dog menace is back. Only this time around, it's not so much dogs that have been affected by rabies; it's raccoons, foxes, bats, coyotes, and even squirrels.

Perhaps no disease is feared as much as rabies. And with good reason. Without treatment, rabies is 100 percent fatal.

In the early days of rabies vaccines, the cure was sometimes as harmful as the disease. The earliest rabies vaccine was made from horse serum and caused allergic reactions in almost everyone who used it. Plus, it was weak. Twenty-three shots were needed. The only muscle big enough to handle that many shots is the abdomen.

Next came a vaccine made from duck embryos. There were fewer reactions to the vaccine, and the regimen dropped down to fourteen shots.

Now, there is HDCV, or human diploid cell vaccine, a five-shot regimen, given in the arm and using a product that rarely causes a sensitivity reaction. Also used is RIG, or rabies immune globulin, a kind of instant vaccine that protects you from the rabies virus while the body is gearing up to manufacture its own antibodies from the HDCV injection. Confused? Here's a look at a rabies exposure, and you can see how the pieces fall into place.

They're at it again. The middle of the day, and those damn raccoons are in the garbage cans. That's it, you say, it's time to get tough with these bandits. You grab a baseball bat and head out to the side of the house. You round the corner and see that it's just one raccoon, and it's staring at you like *you're* the intruder. Why isn't he running away? you wonder as you raise the bat. Just as you're about to let it come crashing down, the raccoon dives from the top of the garbage can and bites you in the arm. Then it growls, spits, falls to the ground, and lunges for your leg. Seconds later, it stumbles across the yard and disappears into the woods.

Treatment

Stunned and badly bleeding, you run back into the house. Was the raccoon rabid? you wonder. Do raccoons even carry rabies? The answer is, overwhelmingly, yes. Raccoons have become the single most important vector in the current rabies epidemic. For example, in Georgia, you are ten times more likely to come in contact with a rabid raccoon than, say, a rabid fox. That's a big change. In the 1950s, the Georgia Department of Public Health paid a bounty for fox heads because they were such heavy transmitters of rabies to dogs. What to do?

1. Remove any clothing the animal's mouth came in contact with and either throw it away or set it aside for solo washing. Then wash the wounds thoroughly with soap and warm water. This is not just busywork. Soap—any bath soap whatsoever— is actually of therapeutic value when it comes to the rabies virus.

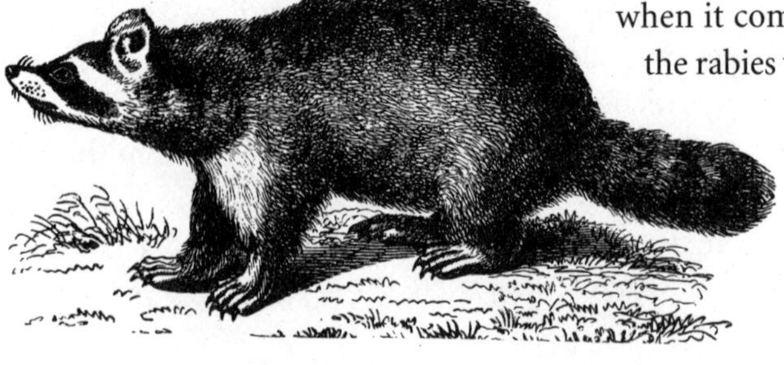

You see, the virus itself is encased in a fatty envelope. Soap dissolves this layer and destroys the virus. In some situations, soap and water washing may nearly be as important as the vaccine.

2. Head to the emergency room and take your checkbook. You have no other choice, other than death. You're going to the emergency room, and you're going to spend lots of money to have your life saved. That's the problem with HDCV: It's extremely expensive. At one time some public health departments paid for rabies vaccines. No more. At $1,000 a pop they couldn't afford to keep doing it. So you'll pay for your life. But come on now, aren't you worth it?

Your wound will probably be cleaned again in the emergency room, and they'll put a rust-colored antiseptic called povidone-iodine around it. Next, you'll get a dose of RIG, or rabies immune globulin. This vaccine provides three weeks' worth of passive immunity. That is, it provides instantaneous protection from the rabies virus by binding it up. Some of the RIG is injected around each wound site and some is injected into the arm. You will also be given your first shot of HDCV, which prompts the body to manufacture antibodies to the rabies virus. And finally, you'll either get a big shot of an antibiotic and/or a prescription for one. That's because animals have trashy mouths that are usually teeming with bacteria.

3. You'll need four more shots of HDCV, so before you leave the emergency room find out where you should go to get them. Some hospitals will send you to your family doctor; some will send you to a public health department. It's not important where you get the shots, it's that you do get them—and get them according to schedule. In rabies parlance, the day you are bitten is called Day Zero. You need additional shots of HDCV on days 3, 7, 14, and 28.

The vaccine is extremely effective. Not a single person has ever developed rabies after treatment with HDCV. But if you think the shots are too much of a hassle and decide to take your chances instead, you're dead.

And the truth is, you will suffer terribly before you die. Maybe a week or two after the bite, you'll come down with what seems like the flu. You will be tired. You may not feel like going to work. You may even experience some pain and itching at the bite site. Within a few more days, you seem constantly thirsty. Yet every time you raise a glass of water to your lips you experience painful spasms in your throat. You find it hard to swallow and you feel agitated, anxious, and apprehensive.

Over the next few more days, you will develop problems walking. Swallowing will continue to be painful. When you are finally admitted to the hospital, they will chain you to the bed and no one will come near you without wearing protective garments. You will be conscious of these things, conscious of your impending death—conscious that you are rabid.

Only two persons have ever recovered from rabies. It's possible you could be the third; if so, you will go down in history. Get the vaccine—even if you have to use a credit card.

How to Avoid Rabies

In our story about the raccoon and the garbage can, there were a few clues that might've tipped you off that the animal was rabid. First off, it was at the garbage cans in the middle of the day. That's unusual behavior. Normally, wild animals wait until nightfall before looking for food. *Any wild animal wandering around during the day is potentially rabid.*

Second, the raccoon didn't run. In other words, it showed no fear. Normally, you'd expect a wild animal to bolt in the face of a human being approaching with a baseball bat. Rabid animals, on the other hand, exhibit a certain crazed boldness. *Any wild animal that seems unafraid of humans is potentially rabid.*

Third, the raccoon attacked. It showed, in other words, unusual aggression. *Any animal that acts in an offensive manner is potentially rabid.*

And finally, the raccoon stumbled into the woods. "Stumbled" is the key here, for the raccoon exhibited symptoms of muscular paralysis. These symptoms could also have included the classic frothing at the mouth, due to paralysis of the throat muscles. *Any animal that appears to be having trouble walking, swallowing, or holding its head up, or that seems "depressed," is potentially rabid.*

Protecting Your Pets from Rabies

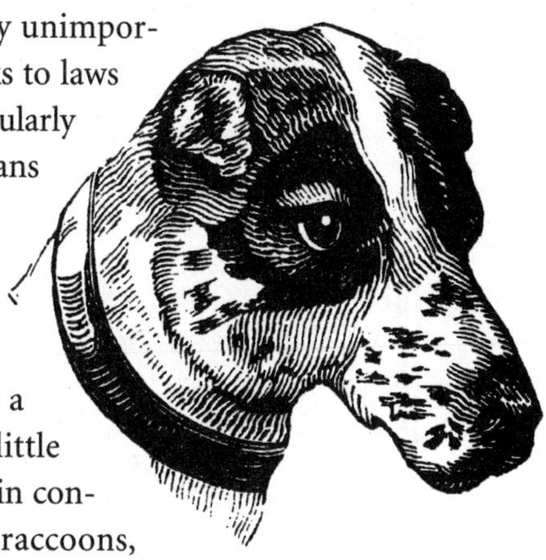

These days, dogs are relatively unimportant transmitters of rabies, thanks to laws that require they be vaccinated regularly against the disease. Regularly means every year. Do it.

Cats are another story. While cat vaccination efforts are under way in some states, regulations are lax in others. And cats have a touch of the wild beast in their little bodies, so they sometimes come in contact with such rabies carriers as raccoons, bats, and skunks. Increasingly, cats are developing rabies. You might feel sorry for a sick stray cat, but let that be as far as it goes. Don't handle it.

Cows can get rabies, too. What's especially dangerous about rabies in livestock is that it's sometimes hard to tell the animal is infected. For example, the main symptom a rabid cow will exhibit is trouble swallowing. This will sometimes prompt a farmer to stick his head inside the cow's mouth to see what's causing the trouble. All the cow needs to do is chomp down on the farmer's head, and he'll wind up with rabies virus injected in the worst possible spot: near the brain and central nervous system.

Rabid horses will, like normal horses, sometimes go berserk, spewing mucus and infectious saliva all over those trying to keep them under control. Even if a rabid horse administers no bite, anyone slathered with its infected saliva is best treated for rabies.

It's a Fact

• It can take years for rabies to develop from a bite. However, most bite victims will develop the disease within a few months.

• Rabies outbreaks move at a rate of about twenty miles a year. The current raccoon epidemic in the northeastern United States started in Florida in the 1960s.

• Mice, rats, moles, and chipmunks don't normally transmit rabies because they are so small they usually die when bitten by another animal. There have been a few cases of rabid squirrels in Connecticut, however.

• Squirrels often exhibit bizzare and aggressive behavior during mating season that might look like rabies. Most likely, it's not. Still, any squirrel bite requires immediate medical attention.

• Rabid skunks are fierce fighters that have been known to kill much larger dogs.

• Spelunkers are at risk of contracting rabies by entering bat-infested caves, because the rabies virus may be carried in the air. Therefore, cave explorers should consider getting prevaccination shots against rabies.

• You can develop rabies without getting a bite. If infectious saliva or a piece of the rabid animal's nervous system tissue gets into the eyes or an open cut, it should be treated as a bite.

• If a bat flies into your face otherwise scratches you, beware: You may have been exposed to rabies. The rule of thumb on bats: If you can't rule out a bite, then you probably need treatment with the rabies vaccine.

Snakes

In a sense, all snakebites are poisonous. Not every snake injects venom, of course, but every snake injects bacteria when it bites. Therefore, *all* snakebites require medical attention, even if that means just getting a tetanus shot.

Of course, the most serious snakebites are those from poisonous snakes. In the United States, poisonous snakes fall into two categories: the elapids, or coral snakes, and the crotalids—rattlesnakes, copperheads, and cottonmouths.

How can you tell if it's a poisonous snake that bit you? In many cases you can't. But there are a few general appearance rules that might lead you to suspect the worst has happened. First, poisonous snakes have distinct heads that flare out from the body at the neck. A nonpoisonous snake looks more like a worm. Poisonous snakes usually have fat, substantial bodies. Nonpoisonous snakes are usually skinny.

Coral Snakes

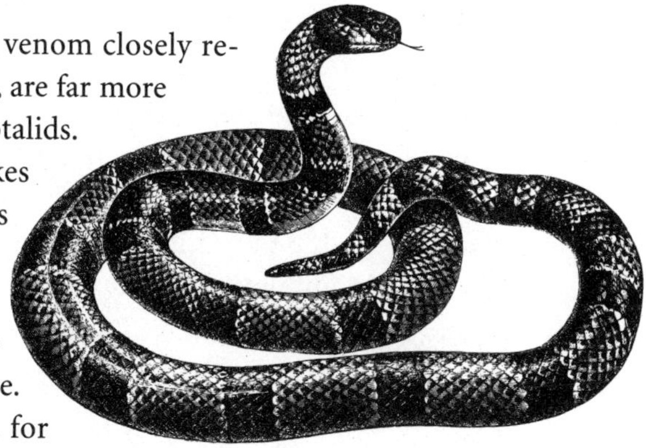

The elapids, whose venom closely resembles that of a cobra, are far more poisonous than the crotalids. Fortunately, coral snakes are shy, timid creatures and seem completely unaware they can kill something three hundred times their own size. We should be grateful for the coral snake's seeming obliviousness to its power. It wants no trouble and usually won't bite unless handled aggressively.

If you *are* bitten by a coral snake, you *must* report to the emergency room or risk death. Coral snake venom attacks the nerves controlling respiration. With crotalids, there is almost always a period of deliberation before the use of antivenin, as some patients get by fine without it. But with coral snakebites, antivenin use is a given.

The bright coloration of the coral snake—red, yellow, and black rings—should be unmistakable. The problem is, there's a nonvenomous king snake that's colored the same way. The key is in the positioning of the colors. When in doubt, remember this rhyme: "Red on yellow, kill a fellow" (coral snake); "red on black, venom lack" (king snake).

Crotalids

A crotalid bite can range from a painful but minor inconvenience all the way to death. It depends on these six things:

- The size of the snake. In general, the bigger the snake the more poisonous it is likely to be. That isn't always true, though. Some very big snakes are also very old and may have shriveled venom glands.
- The species of crotalid. In general, rattlesnakes are the most poisonous, with cottonmouths not far behind. Copperheads are considered the least poisonous. However, there is significant variation within the rattlesnake family. For example, the pygmy rattler—technically in the genus *Sistrurus*—is mildly poisonous.
- The age and health of the victim. The very young, very old, and very sick are most at risk from snakebites.
- The site of the bite. It's better to get bitten in muscle or fat tissue, as the venom is then absorbed more slowly. The worst place to take a bite is directly into a blood vessel.
- The emotional state of the patient *and* the snake. Emotion is

your enemy in a snakebite, on both sides of the equation. An emotional snake injects more venom, and an emotional victim's fast heart rate spreads that venom around the body faster.

- The depth of the wound. Sometimes, a snake's fangs will just scratch the skin, injecting only a small amount of venom. Deep wounds are the most dangerous.

Crotalid venom can do disgusting things to human flesh, because the venom penetrates the walls of small blood vessels. The swelling that results can be so severe that the tissue around the bite bursts open under pressure. As the hemorrhaging continues, the crotalid wound turns purple, red, and black. Needless to say, the wound is extremely painful.

Hospital Treatment

A bad-looking wound, in and of itself, is not an indication to use antivenin. Instead, it's the symptoms that occur *away* from the bite site that cause the most concern. If a snakebite victim complains of nausea, dizziness, or tingling sensations, especially atop the scalp, it's a sign of a serious envenomation. That's the time to use antivenin.

Normally, these serious symptoms will occur—if they're going to occur—within six hours of a snakebite. But they may not come on gradually. A snakebite victim can be perfectly fine, save for local swelling and pain, for several hours after a bite, and then, without warning, can become extremely sick. That's why *all poisonous snakebites must be observed in the emergency room for a minimum of six hours.*

During that observation period, the hospital staff will measure the swelling's progression, do some blood and urine testing, and perhaps test to see if you're allergic to antivenin in case they need to use it. That's an important consideration, as the antivenin is made from horse serum, a potent inducer of allergic reactions.

Treatment in the Wilderness

1. Keep the victim calm. Remember, emotion is the enemy in a snakebite situation.

2. If possible, keep the bite area at a level slightly below the heart.

3. Don't put any ice on the wound. Ice freezes and damages the tissue.

4. Sucking on the wound is dangerous, because the venom could get into small cuts inside the mouth. Use an extractor. These devices fit over the bite area and, when pulled on, exert pressure that may help remove some venom. Don't count on this as a cure-all, however.

5. A loose tourniquet is okay, but the key here is *loose.* Don't cut off blood flow to the bite area.

6. Get help as fast as possible.

Your best bet, of course, is prevention. Know where snakes like to hide—in stone walls, tree trunks, piles of brush, garbage, lumber, and logs; in open fields; and along desert roads at night—and avoid these areas! If you can't, wear heavy boots.

When in the wilderness carry a snake stick with you at all times and use it—not to beat up snakes but rather to rustle the brush in front of you, so as to scare off or reveal any serpents before you step on them. Use a snake stick before stepping over obstructions, as well. The rule is: If you can't see what's on the other side, check it first with your stick.

If you encounter a snake, back off slowly and let it get away. These are dangerous creatures when cornered, and you should leave them alone.

Never go for a swim in the wilderness unless you have checked the area for snakes. Snakes can swim, and in the south, cottonmouths (water moccasins) prefer to lounge on the banks of rivers, streams, and ponds, as well as on tree limbs.

It's a Fact

• The largest poisonous snakes in the United States are the eastern diamondback rattlers. They can grow seven to nine feet long. Second largest is the western diamondback rattler. The latter cause more snakebite fatalities in the United States than any other type. The most deadly rattlesnake in the world is the cascavel, found in South America; its venom is more powerful than a cobra's.

• With the exception of zoo specimens, there are no poisonous snakes in the United States that are colored green.

• Riding across the desert at night? Don't get out of your car for any reason. Desert-dwelling snakes gravitate toward asphalt because it's warm.

• Rattlesnakes can spit venom into the eyes. This will cause irritation but not blindness.

• The Santa Catalina rattlesnake has one unusual characteristic: It has no rattler.

• Cottonmouths, or water moccasins, have venom nearly as potent as that of a rattlesnake and can be very aggressive if cornered.

• Copperheads inflict the least poisonous bites. Frequently, they require no treatment with antivenin.

• Severed snake heads may bite for up to one hour after being cut. Never touch a snake that's been killed.

• Snakes are deaf, but their tongues may enable them to "hear" things.

• King snakes feed on rattlesnakes and appear to be immune to rattlesnake venom.

• About fifteen thousand cans of rattlesnake meat are sold in the United States each year.

• Some poisonous snakes in the United States are considered nonpoisonous because their fangs aren't positioned to inject venom. These include the black-banded snake, the lyre snake, and the Texas cat-eyed snake.

Fish

And you thought all you had to worry about at the beach was a sunburn? Yes, it's true; you can't even go swimming without possibly running into a poisonous creature.

Jellyfish and Portuguese Man-of-Wars

Those of us living in the United States have little to worry about if we're stung by a jellyfish or a man-of-war, save for pain. But take note: The pain can be excruciating. These ocean-dwelling creatures have special cells called nematocysts that are the equivalent of poison spear launchers. Brush up against them, and out zooms a poisonous thread. With the Portuguese man-of-war, the thread is barbed and spiked and can therefore be difficult to remove from the skin.

It's a Fact

- The largest jellyfish in the world, the sea blubber, has a body six feet across and tentacles up to two hundred feet long.
- The most deadly jellyfish is the sea wasp, found off the Australian coast. A sting from the sea wasp can kill a human within an hour.
- The body of the jellyfish is made of jelly; the body of the Portuguese man-of-war is a fleshy bladder filled with gas.
- Jellyfish evaporate so quickly, once washed up onto the beach, because they are 99 percent water. However, even dried-up jellyfish and man-of-wars can inflict nasty stings.
- The Portuguese man-of-war's venom is chemically related to the cobra's.

Treatment

Removing the poisonous threads is really the most bothersome part of treating a jellyfish injury. Try a clean knife edge and be sure to wear gloves. But first, irrigate the wound area with seawater and vinegar. Don't touch it without gloves and don't rub it. The pain may linger for some time, and you might try a local anesthetic or even an oral anti-inflammatory like ibuprofen or naproxen. Hydrocortisone cream may also alleviate some of the irritation. Pain from the wound will gradually decrease but may persist for days after the sting. Watch for signs of infection: increased warmth, redness, and pain to the touch. If these occur see a doctor.

On occasion, the reaction to a jellyfish sting might be a more severe allergic one. Basically, if you see anything other than a local reaction—that is pain, redness, and swelling at the site of the sting—you need to see a doctor, and fast. Some of the reactions might include a more extensive rash, shortness of breath, nausea, dizziness, and headache.

Lionfish and Catfish

The peacocks of the aquarium world, lionfish belong to a family of poisonous fish that includes the deadly stonefish. Usually, an exposure to the lionfish occurs when an aquarium owner reaches in to clean the tank and the fish's poison-filled fins brush up against the skin. The result is immediate pain. Later, nausea and weakness may develop.

Treatment

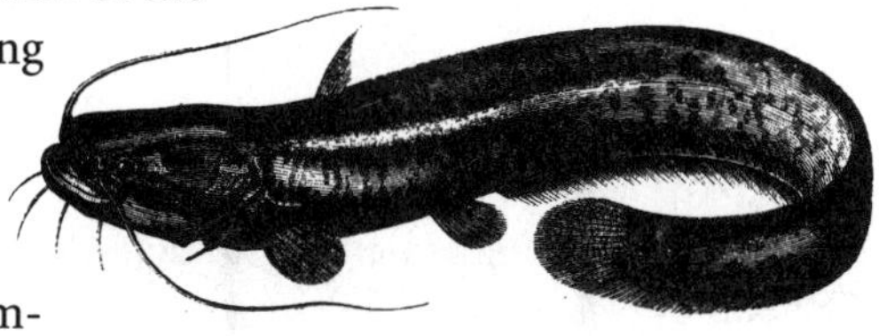

Treatment is easy. The venom of the lionfish is heat labile, meaning it's destroyed at a high temperature. So, immediately after the sting, wash the wound area well and then immerse it in a pan of water as hot as you can stand, perhaps as high as 110 to 115 degrees Fahrenheit. Use common sense here. *Don't use water that is at or near the boiling point, or you will inflict serious injury on the skin and underlying tissues.* Any pieces of the fish remaining in the skin should be removed, and this is an excellent opportunity to get a tetanus booster if you need one. Antibiotics may also be needed to prevent infection.

Catfish stings are handled the same way, but they are generally less serious than those from the lionfish.

Lizards and Toads

Gila Monster

The gila monster (pronounced *hee-la*) is the only poisonous lizard found in the United States. This brightly colored, chunky creature spends most of its time underground, so you are highly unlikely to encounter a gila unless you go looking for one.

Don't. Gila monsters are like a cross between a pit bull and a poisonous snake. They're not aggressive, but once they bite they hang on. In fact, they're so tenacious they sometimes have to be torn from the skin.

It's a Fact

- If you kill a gila monster in the wild you have violated the law. It's a protected species in the four states in which it's found: Utah, California, Arizona, Nevada.
- In the hottest parts of Arizona, gila monsters may spend up to 98 percent of their lives undercover.

Treatment

The gila's venom is chemically related to the cobra's, but serious envenomations by the lizard are rare. Instead, it's usually more of a wound problem. At the hospital, the wound will be thoroughly cleaned and disinfected and a tetanus shot will be given. There is no specific antidote for gila monster poisonings, nor is one generally needed. If you're bitten in the wild, do not use ice on the wound. Instead, place the wounded area at or near the level of the heart and get medical attention.

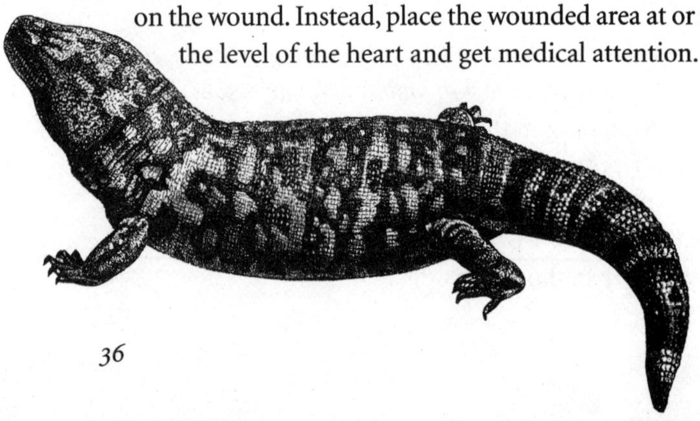

Toads

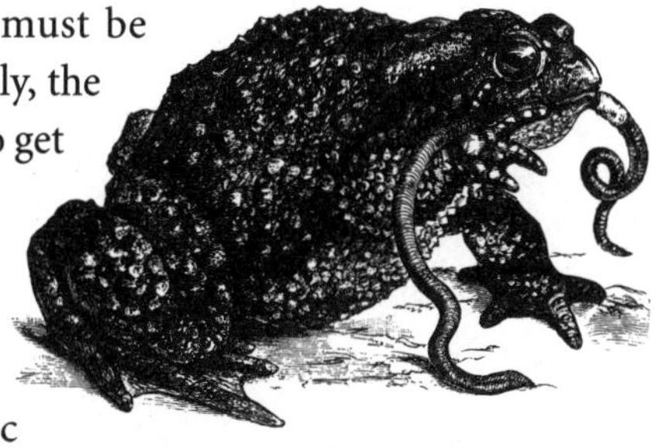

Poisonous toads? You must be kidding! Afraid not. Actually, the average person isn't likely to get poisoned by contact with a toad, but they are a serious danger for pets. The problem is, toads secrete poisons that act like the toxic heart drug digoxin. The eating of a toad by a dog—or even holding the toad in its mouth or drinking water from a dish where a toad has sat for some time—can poison and even kill the canine.

Needless to say, humans shouldn't eat toads either. After handling a toad, always wash your hands thoroughly and don't put them anywhere near your eyes until they're clean. Toad secretions are extremely irritating to mucus membranes. All toad ingestions—whether by a pet or a human being—are a medical emergency.

2

The Yard

Look beneath the surface of any well-tended yard and you'll find a killing field of chemicals. Most of these products are, in fact, quite toxic to humans and pets, but for home use they are usually only available in dilute solutions. Thus, with the exception of snail and slug killers, small exposures to yard products usually result in only minor problems. It's a different story with plants. While non-toxic varieties abound, nature has packed some plants with highly potent and even occasionally deadly toxins. A word to the wise (and we'll remind you again later)—*know the name of every plant you've got in your yard*—just in case.

Insecticides

Pliny the Elder, a Roman author, had it all figured out when it came to pest control. He recommended having a bare-breasted "nubile virgin" cruise the garden grounds. This ritual, according to Pliny, caused caterpillars to fall to the ground.

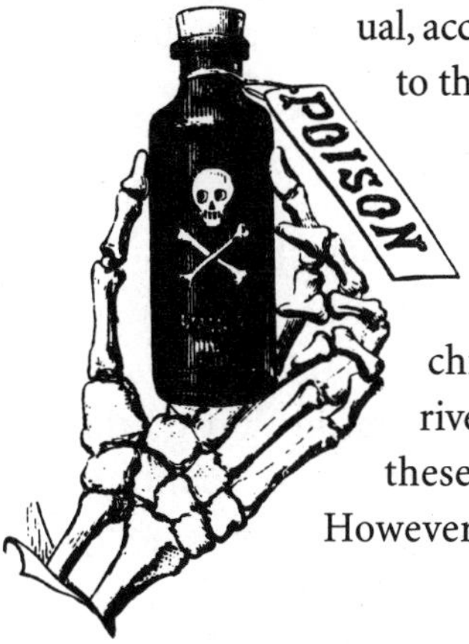

Ah, for old-time pest control! These days we make do with a list of most unsexy substitutes, pesticides that range from natural products distilled from chrysanthemum flowers to chemicals derived from Nazi nerve gas. And yes, many of these chemicals are extremely poisonous. However, home exposures tend to be small. So while there's always the possibility of a problem, it rarely happens unless there's massive misuse of the product.

Many gardeners who are looking for the least of the evils, when it comes to pesticides, have found it in insecticidal soaps. These products make unappetizing the juicy leaves of your perennials and annuals, but if accidentally ingested by a human or a pet they rarely cause anything more significant than minor vomiting. We are concerned here with the next step up: chemical insecticides. Among these the pyrethrins tend to be the least toxic, the organophosphates the most poisonous.

Pyrethrins

Mum's the word—as in chrysanthemum, that is. The pyrethrins, derived from these autumnal flowers, have been used in pest control since the first century B.C. Their popularity waned somewhat during the golden age of chemical pesticides in the 1940s and 1950s, but they're more popular than ever now, thanks to the realization that pesticides like DDT terribly interrupt the ecosystem.

"Natural" does not necessarily mean safe for human beings. But in the case of pyrethrins and their synthetic cousins the pyrethroids, poisonings tend to be mild. The exception is with massive exposures—such as might occur in a crop-dusting operation—or in those with severe asthma, when life-threatening bronchospasms can occur.

Treatment

Pyrethrin products include Spectracide Bug Stop, Enforcer Flea Fogger, and Hot Shot Fogger and Ant and Roach Killer. As you might expect with a plant-derived product, the chief symptoms of pyrethrin poisoning are allergic: a scratchy throat, itchy eyes, a bit of coughing, and perhaps a short spell of vomiting. That's usually it. Piperonyl butoxide, an insecticide commonly found in tandem with pyrethrins, is also low in toxicity.

The imperative with any pesticide exposure is fresh air, and that's usually all you need for a pyrethrin poisoning. But if wheezing continues or tightness in the chest develops, go to the emergency room. Asthmatics can develop life-threatening symptoms from pyrethrin exposures.

Pyrethrins and pets are a dangerous combination. If you've ever had a cat who was "flea-dipped" at the vet's and then later developed seizures, you have some idea of what pyrethrins can do to small animals. Dogs and cats are far more sensitive to pyrethrins than humans. (Experienced vets, by the way, know how to prevent a flea-dip seizure.)

That said, numerous flea and tick products meant to be sprayed on the coats of pets contain pyrethrins. The key to safe use of these products is to keep the exposure to a minimum. Never spray a concentrated amount on your pet, and never spray any flea and tick killer on a puppy or kitten. They're more susceptible to pyrethrin poisoning than an adult dog or cat.

What's a pyrethroid? When it comes to pest control, chemists can never leave well enough alone. There are now many pyrethroids—synthetic pyrethrins—on the market. Usually, their names will end with the suffix "thrin." Permethrin is one example; another is the powerful decamethrin.

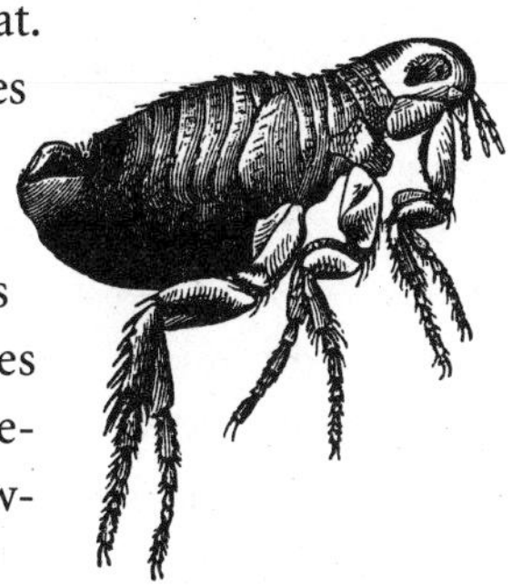

Carbamates and Organophosphates

Choose your poison. Carbamates include Baygon, Sevin, and many others; Diazinon, Dichlorvos, Dursban, Malathion, and many others are organophosphates.

These insecticides inhibit the breakdown of a chemical called acetylcholine. Acetylcholine keeps our nervous systems working. Every time you pick up a pencil, sip a glass of water, or even think, acetylcholine is helping you do it. But nerve cells need a slight rest between each electrical impulse, and that's where acetylcholinesterase comes in. ACHE, as it's called, breaks down acetylcholine just after it interacts with a nerve cell. That gives the nerve cell its needed moment of rest. Then the next batch of acetylcholine comes along, and the nerve is restimulated.

By preventing the breakdown of acetylcholine, these insecticides cause the nerve cells to become so highly stimulated that they become, in effect, *paralyzed* with stimulation. It's almost like the nerves are being chemically electrocuted.

Obviously, this can lead to significant problems, and organophosphates in particular can be deadly. The symptoms these insecticides produce are known as SLUDGE, medical shorthand for lots of fluids oozing from lots of places. The acronym stands for Salivation, Lacrimation (tearing), Urination, Diarrhea (or Diaphoresis, which is sweating), Gastrointestinal effects, and Emesis (another word for vomiting).

Treatment

Of course you need to be careful when using an organophosphate or carbamate insecticide at home, but what's the likelihood that the typical small home exposure—a slight inhalation or a couple of drops ingested—will result in SLUDGE symptoms? The answer is: low. Most anytime you call a poison center about such an exposure you'll be told to do nothing but watch for symptoms: no ipecac syrup, no immediate trip to the hospital. Just observe.

It's a different story with a substantial exposure—substantial, in this case, defined as anything more than, say, a taste of insecticide. These kinds of poisonings need immediate medical attention. Don't induce vomiting, just go to the emergency room.

Chlorinated Hydrocarbons

This group of insecticides, including aldrin, dieldrin, heptachlor, and lindane, reads like a hall of fame for environmental disaster: DDT, chlordane, mirex. In chemistry, anytime you chlorinate anything you're asking for trouble. And the problem with these insecticides—aside from the fact they're rather nonselective in their killing—is that they persist in the environment.

Because of their danger, many of these insecticides have been banned, and the most likely way you'd be exposed to one in the home is through a pest control company that has a special license to use them; through the use of the pharmaceutical product lindane, a treatment for lice; or if you live near an agricultural field that employs aerial spraying.

Treatment

The chlorinated hydrocarbons affect the nervous system. Thus, in a toxic exposure, symptoms could range from minor (dizziness, headache) to severe (seizures and death). Again, you will most likely be asked to observe for symptoms rather than rush off to the emergency room, unless there's been a substantial ingestion. Don't use ipecac syrup.

How long should you stay away from a house that has been treated for termites?

Unfortunately, there's no exact answer to that question. If you have small children or an infant in the house, plan to stay away until odors dissipate—perhaps up to forty-eight hours. Otherwise, plan on a twenty-four-hour hiatus. It's not that the odors themselves are poisonous, but they're annoying and distressing. And with infants—whose everyday existence includes many of the symptoms of SLUDGE—it's hard to tell sometimes what's normal and what isn't. Still, the likelihood of developing insecticide poisoning from a termite treatment seems

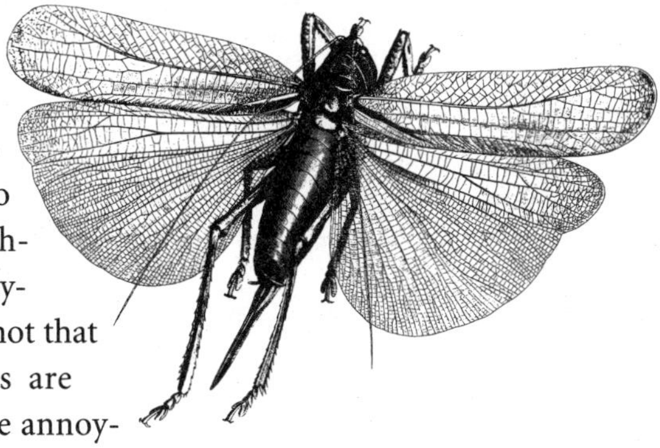

It's a Fact

• Perhaps the most famous case of organophosphate poisoning occurred in the 1930s during Prohibition when a bootlegger diluted an alcohol-containing tonic called Ginger Jake with a furniture finisher called Lyndol. The bootlegger didn't realize it, but he had contaminated some of the Ginger Jake with an organophosphate called TOCP. At least five thousand people were poisoned by the drink, many developing permanent weakness and paralysis of the legs. The distinctive gait that resulted inspired several hit songs, including "The Jake Leg Blues."

• Fatty foods increase the absorption of chlorinated hydrocarbons. Avoid foods like milk after an exposure.

• Organophosphates, carbamates, and chlorinated hydrocarbons can all be absorbed through the skin and the eyes and through inhalation. Any large-scale exposure to the skin should be immediately and thoroughly washed off with soap and water. For the eyes, skip the soap and rinse the eyes well with lukewarm water for a good fifteen minutes. Also, take note: The human scrotum is one of the worst places to spill a chemical because it's loaded with blood vessels. Never continue to wear a chemical-soaked pair of pants, especially when dealing with insecticides.

• The difference between organophosphates and carbamates is that the former are considered permanent disablers of ACHE, while the latter only temporarily disable the enzyme.

• Severe organophosphate poisoning can be reversed with the antidote Protopam (2-PAM).

• Parathion, the first organophosphate, was discovered by the Germans in the 1940s during research for the Nazi chemical war agents sarin and tabun.

• Insect resistance to DDT exploded after its introduction in the 1940s. By 1976, more than two hundred insect species were resistant to DDT.

continued

- Want to try the pagan method of pest control? Pray to Flora, as the Romans did. She's the goddess of mildew.
- Paris green, the first chemical insecticide, was made from arsenic. Initially, it was used in France to scare humans from stealing grapes.
- Boric acid, sometimes used to control roaches, has low toxicity. In most cases, a lick of boric acid will cause no symptoms, but bluish-green vomiting and diarrhea are possible.
- Talk about a lack of prescience. The Swiss chemist who discovered DDT won a Nobel Prize for the accomplishment. His name was Paul Hermann Müller.

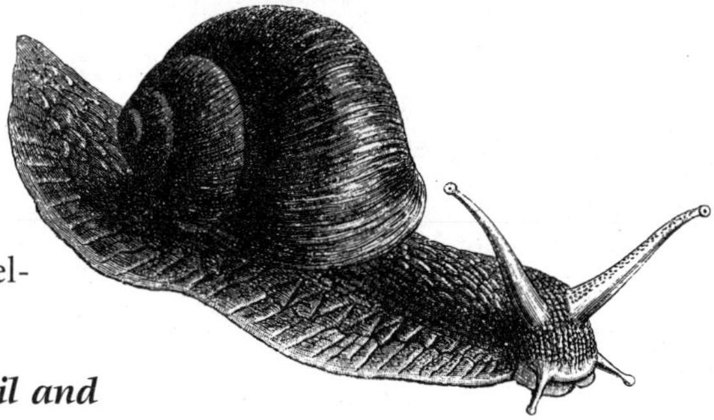

low. I recently had my house treated and never left. It stunk, to be sure. But we never developed any problems.

Metaldehyde Snail and Slug Killers

Snails are some tough customers to kill. The proof: metaldehyde slug killers—Deadline Bullets, Bug-Geta—are one of the most toxic substances you'll find in the yard. Less than a teaspoonful of a slug killer containing metaldehyde can kill a child or pet. Metaldehyde causes severe cramping, diarrhea, and vomiting. Toxicity can progress to seizures and a coma as well. Ingestion of a snail and slug killer is a medical emergency. Do not use ipecac syrup. Call the poison center and prepare to go to the hospital.

DEET Insect Repellent

Don't eat DEET. In fact, don't even apply DEET very often; it can be absorbed through the skin and over time can produce severe toxicity. Always use the weakest DEET product you can get away with, as those with a high concentration have been associated with seizures —even when just applied to the skin. What's a high concentration of DEET? Well, for serious jungle adventurers, 50 percent DEET solutions are available. But for children, some products now contain as little as 5 percent. Keep the DEET concentration under 10 percent, and you should be safe.

It's a Fact

• Consider insect repellents with DEET "occasional-use" products. They should not be slathered on every day, as toxicity could result.

• It's safer to wear more clothes than apply more DEET. Covering large areas of the body with the repellent is more likely to result in toxicity. Another idea: Apply the DEET to your clothes instead of the skin.

• Report any oral ingestion of DEET to the poison center. However, a taste of one of the low-concentration products is not likely to result in symptoms.

• DEET stands for N,N-diethyl-meta-toluamide. Now you know why we prefer to call it DEET.

Herbicides

Paraquat and Diquat

Many of us first heard about paraquat in 1978, after it was used to kill marijuana crops in Mexico. The concern back then was that contaminated marijuana would find its way onto the streets and start killing people. Thankfully, that didn't happen. Paraquat is one of the most toxic substances ever developed; a tablespoonful of paraquat concentrate is enough to kill an adult.

Ingestions of paraquat—even a swallow—can cause kidney failure. If that doesn't kill the victim, a lung condition called pulmonary fibrosis, which develops over the course of a week after the poisoning, probably will.

Diquat, which is kind of like paraquat "lite," is the home version of this poison. It's also highly toxic. But most home weed killers, such as Spectracide, contain only a small amount of diquat—some as low as 0.25 percent. Even at that low concentration, a few ounces of a commercial product can result in severe irritation and even ulcerations of the throat and digestive tract.

> **It's a Fact**
>
> • While it's not available for home use, paraquat can sometimes be found on large farms in the South, where it's used to make cotton harvesting easier by killing the leaves and exposing the bolls.
>
> • Paraquat is not easily absorbed through the skin, unless the skin is abraded or the affected area is a blood-rich tissue like the scrotum, which is permeable to almost any chemical.
>
> • Sunlight deactivates paraquat. So once it's sprayed on plants it breaks down.

Treatment

If a child has been around a diquat-containing weed killer and suddenly screams his mouth is burning, you might suspect an herbicidal ingestion and get him to the emergency room. Death from home products can occur if enough is ingested, but the burning sensation inside the mouth probably limits exposures to a swallow. Diquat in the eyes is dangerous: Rinse the eyes thoroughly with lukewarm water for fifteen to thirty minutes and plan to have them examined. Do the same for a skin exposure.

Chlorophenoxy Herbicides

Many "weed and feed" products—Spectracide Weed Stop, WeedBGon—contain chlorophenoxy herbicides, and small ingestions tend to cause immediate irritation. For small ingestions, dilute by drinking a glass of water and expect vomiting to occur. Large ingestions—a rare event—can cause death. So if you're unsure of the amount, let the emergency room handle it.

Glyphosate and Trifluralin

It's all relative, of course, but the safest weed killers are those containing glyphosate (Round-Up) and trifluralin (Preen 'N' Green). That's not to say these are nonpoisonous. In small doses, both irritate the throat and mouth, sometimes resulting in vomiting (probably more likely with glyphosate than trifluralin).

Treatment

For small ingestions of either, rinse out the mouth using the "swish and spit" method. Follow this up with a glass of water, juice, or milk. Vomiting may occur. If it does, rinse the mouth again. There is no need to seek medical treatment unless the vomiting is severe.

For eye exposures, rinse for up to thirty minutes with lukewarm water. Unless there's extreme distress, allow another thirty minutes to elapse *after* you've finished rinsing before making a decision on further medical treatment. This gives the eyes a chance to recover from the rinsing you've done.

For the skin, wash thoroughly with soap and water.

It's a Fact

• The toxicity of Agent Orange, the infamous herbicide mixture used to defoliate the jungles during the Vietnam War, was more due to the dioxin that commonly occurred as a contaminant during its manufacture. Dioxin, or TCDD, is one of the most toxic substances known to man.

Plant Foods and Dirt

Fertilizers

Let's move now from killing plants to nurturing them. Home fertilizers are, in general, weak nitrogen-containing compounds that when swallowed might cause some vomiting but little else. Sure, if you've got someone who's making a meal out of a bag of Miracle-Gro, symptoms might be more severe: profuse vomiting, perhaps burns in the mouth, maybe even methemoglobinemia, a poisonous blood condition. But for small ingestions, just give a glass of water or juice. Seek medical help for severe vomiting. For fertilizer in the eyes or on the skin, rinse thoroughly with lukewarm water.

> **It's a Fact**
>
> • The lime you put on your lawn is corrosive: ingestions can damage the mouth and throat. Rinse out the mouth with water. Blistered tissue, problems swallowing, and excessive drooling might indicate tissue damage.

Dirt

Yeah, people eat dirt. Clearly, something has gone awry with these individuals, because dirt is neither tasty nor particularly good for you. In fact, it could be bad for you. For one thing, it might contain parasites or bacteria—animals, after all, use the earth as their toilet. Second, because the texture of dirt is, shall we say, a bit dense, a substantial ingestion of dirt can clog up the intestines.

But the common mouthful-of-dirt ingestion you usually see in children is not a big deal. Rinse the mouth thoroughly and give a glass of juice or water. If you see symptoms that resemble food poisoning—cramping, diarrhea, fever—consult a doctor.

Bagged dirt—potting soil, composted manure, topsoil, peat moss—is probably *less* dangerous than the dirt in your backyard because it may be sanitized before it's packaged. That lessens the likelihood of bacterial poisoning.

Poisonous Plants

First of all, know your plants. Don't find yourself in this situation: Your child has eaten some berries off a bush in your yard. You don't know the name of the bush. You don't know how many berries were eaten. You call the local poison control center, hoping they can help. "My child ate these purple berries," you say. "I don't know what they are."

The bad news is, the poison center can't tell you what they are either. So the first thing you're going to do after reading this chapter is go out into your yard and do a plant inventory. Find out what you have. If you can't identify it, take a clipping to a local nursery and see if they can help you. Once you know what you've got, make a list and don't lose it. If you have a plant name, the poison center can almost always help you.

How poisonous are they? Without a doubt, there are some deadly plants out there. But practically speaking, many poisonous plants are easily tolerated if the exposure is small.

Oxalates

A case in point is those plants that contain oxalates. These small, irritating crystals get released into the mouth when the plant is chewed, causing intense pain and inflammation. Fortunately, the pain is so intense that large ingestions are rare.

How can you identify an oxalate-containing plant? For the most part, you can't. But some of these plants *do* have a common characteristic: heart-shaped leaves that can sometimes be huge. They include anthurium, caladium, elephant's ear, monstera, philodendron, taro, and xanthosoma.

Oxalate plants with less-pronounced leaves include agave, arum, begonia (some), calla lily, dieffenbachia (dumbcane), jack-in-the-pulpit, pothos, shamrocks, and skunk cabbage.

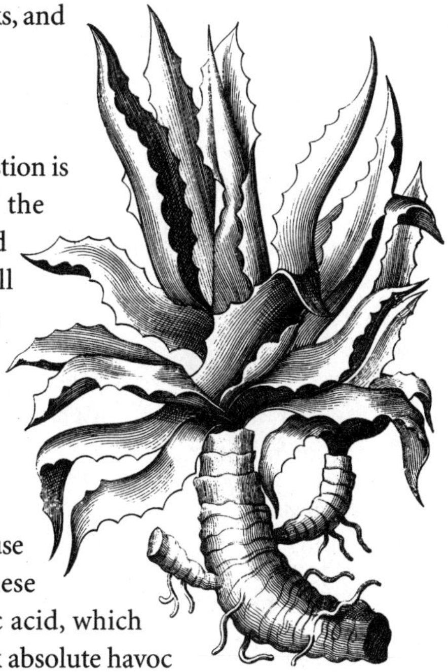

Treatment

Treating a small oxalate ingestion is easy. Wipe out the inside of the mouth using a soft, milk-soaked cloth. Then administer a small glass of milk. Finally, if there's persistent pain, pull a Popsickle out of the freezer. Sucking on one of these usually does the trick.

Warning: Some oxalic acid–containing plants *won't* cause mouth pain. That's because these contain *soluble* forms of oxalic acid, which can get into the body and wreak absolute havoc on the kidneys, heart, and liver. Rhubarb leaves and sorrel contain soluble oxalic acid. Rhubarb stalks also contain soluble oxalic acid, but much less than in the leaves. In fact, it's oxalic acid that gives rhubarb stalks their distinctive tang.

Skin Irritants

Many plants irritate the skin and eyes. However, for most such exposures, the remedy is simple: water. Soap doesn't hurt either, if you're dealing with a skin exposure. The point is, these exposures tend to be mild, and a good ten-minute eye rinse or skin flush should take care of most symptoms. Eating one of these plants might cause vomiting; give a glass of fluid and observe. Irritant plants include aster, black-eyed susan, bleeding heart, chrysanthemum, cleome, daisy, fig tree, gas plant, globe thistle, hyacinth, primrose, tulip, and verbena.

Poison Ivy, Oak, and Sumac

These plants contain a powerfully irritating substance called urushiol, which causes intense irritation, itching, and swelling. Now remember: It's the urushiol—the plant liquid—that causes the spread of the poison ivy, oak, or sumac rash. It's *not* necessarily the liquid that drains from the blisters caused by the rash, unless that liquid contains some urushiol that hasn't yet reacted with the skin. Therefore, once a case of poison ivy, oak, or sumac has settled in, the person with the rash is usually noninfectious. Clothing is another matter. Because some of the urushiol may have rubbed onto the victim's clothes, it's important to wash them thoroughly *and separately* from other pieces of clothing.

Treatment

Cases of poison ivy, oak, and sumac can range from an irritating itch to a debilitating rash. It really depends on individual sensitivity. For all cases, wash the body thoroughly with soap and water. If a rash appears, use an oral antihistamine (like diphenhydramine), as well as something on the rash itself: calamine, hydrocortisone cream, or Domeboro soaks.

See a doctor if large, globular blisters develop or if the rash hits a sensitive area, such as the eyes or genitals.

Gastrointestinal Irritants

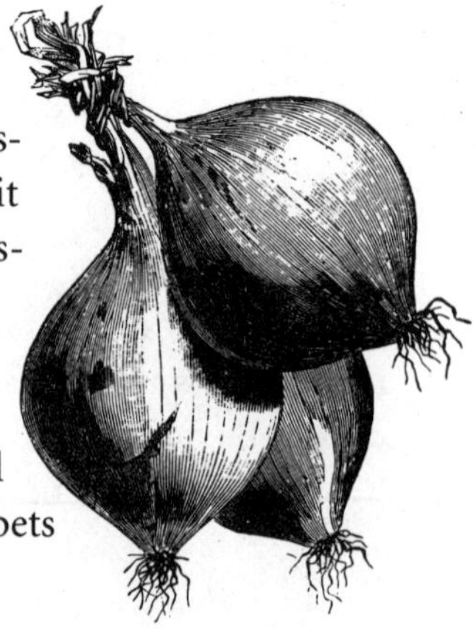

BULBS. Let's hope, you will never be invited to a dinner where someone has mistaken amaryllis bulbs for onions. But it happens. And the results might be mistaken as a *severe* insult to the cook: abdominal cramping, diarrhea, vomiting, and weakness that could persist for a few days. In general, ingestion of one bulb will not result in serious symptoms, but all bets are off on a multibulb meal. Some of these plants include allium (all species), amaryllis (lilies), hyacinth, iris (many species), lily of the Nile (agapanthus), narcissus (daffodils), snowdrop, and star of Bethlehem.

GREEN POTATOES. Almost every poisonous plant, no matter by what mechanism it will eventually kill you (if it *will* kill you), starts off by irritating the stomach and intestines. But there are a few plants in which gastrointestinal irritation is the main and sometimes only toxicity—like green potatoes.

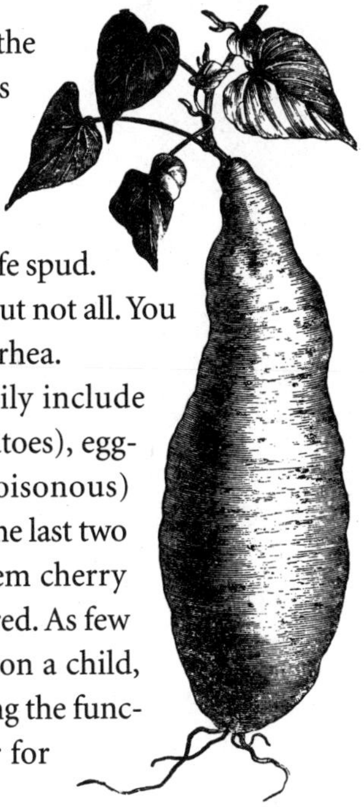

Yes, potato poisonings happen, due to the chemical solanine. So never eat potatoes that have a green cast to them or you may become sick. Never eat potato sprouts or "berries." And don't be fooled into thinking that a cooked green potato is a safe spud. Cooking will remove some of the toxins, but not all. You can still wind up with cramping and diarrhea.

Other members of the solanine family include tomatoes (but it's okay to eat green tomatoes), eggplant, and the inedible (and highly poisonous) Jerusalem cherry and Japanese lanterns. The last two plants develop attractive berries. Jerusalem cherry berries start off green and turn a blazing red. As few as three or four of these berries can poison a child, both by irritating the stomach and affecting the function of the heart. Call the poison center for advice if an ingestion occurs.

Other plants that primarily cause gastrointestinal problems include aloe vera, boxwood, the chinaberry tree (extremely toxic; fewer than ten berries will produce severe symptoms), delphinium, English Ivy, four o'clock, hydrangea, lupine (plus headache and dizziness possible, but all symptoms usually mild), and wisteria. Reactions to these can range from mild cramping, diarrhea, and vomiting with a plant like aloe vera all the way to extremely severe symptoms with the chinaberry tree.

ACORNS. Obviously, squirrels have strong stomachs. Otherwise, they'd never be able to munch on acorns, which contain tannins. You can tell from the first bitter bite of a tannin-containing plant (another such plant is the poinciana) that it's not good to eat. In the intestines, those irritating properties result in severe cramping, vomiting, and diarrhea. Eating just one acorn is enough to cause symptoms, but small ingestions can sometimes be handled at home. The leaves from the oak tree contain tannins, as well.

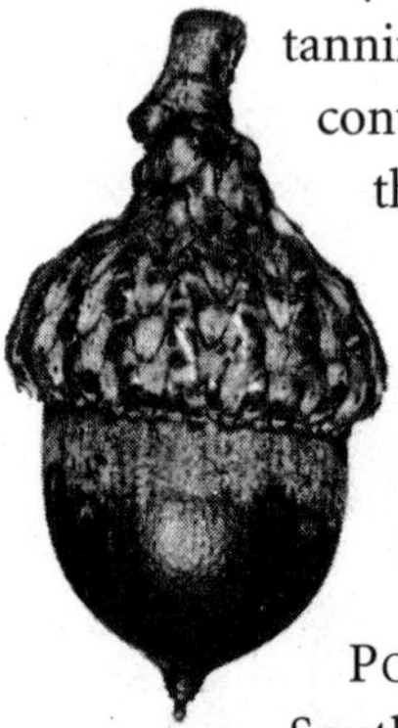

POKEWEED. How about a bowl of poke salad? In the South—God only knows why—countryfolk prepare a dish from pokeweed greens called poke salad. No matter what anybody tells you, don't eat it. Pokeweed contains toxins that cause severe cramping, vomiting, and diarrhea. You can cook these toxins out—and that's precisely what folks try to do—but it takes two separate "waters" to do it. The problem is, even when cooked, poke salad still contains a substance that may damage blood cells.

The most common poisoning scenario with pokeweed comes from ingesting improperly cooked greens or some of its luscious-looking purple berries. In a small child, even a few of these berries could cause an upset stomach, though it takes a good handful before treatment is recommended.

Fortunately, pokeberries taste so bad that most children will avoid eating large amounts. As for poke salad, cooking isn't the answer. While it can reduce the immediate toxicity of pokeweed, it does nothing to change its possible long-term effect on blood cells. Avoid it.

HORSE CHESTNUTS. Chestnuts roasting on an open fire . . . ? Pity those who mistake horse chestnuts for the Christmas kind made famous by Bing Crosby. Horse chestnuts contain aesculin, a chemical that affects the blood and severely irritates the stomach. If a number of horse chestnuts are eaten, stupor and paralysis could result. Horse chestnut ingestions are usually treated in the emergency room.

CLEMATIS. A pretty, vinous perennial with white, purple, or mauve flowers, often found on mailboxes, clematis contains a substance that burns up the mouth so badly that most ingestions are limited to a small taste. Treating a small clematis ingestion is easy: Wash and rinse out the mouth well and give a Popsicle. If blisters begin appearing inside the mouth, or if there's pain or trouble swallowing, see a doctor immediately. Other plants with a toxicity similar to clematis include buttercups, which taste terrible, and marsh marigold.

PLANTS IN THE TOBACCO FAMILY. The lobelia or cardinal flower, a plant in the tobacco family, contains lobeline, a compound similar to nicotine but much less potent. It's unlikely a small ingestion of a cardinal flower plant will result in toxicity, but if you see vomiting it's a sign that more dangerous things might be on the way—like a rise in blood pressure.

Possibly more dangerous are plants which contain cytisine, another nicotinelike compound. Again, vomiting and changes in heart rate and blood pressure, as well as seizures, can occur with large doses. But small ingestions probably aren't a problem. Cytisine-containing plants include the wild indigo, false indigo, Kentucky coffee tree, and Spanish broom. Be more careful with ingestions of the golden chain tree, mescal bean saphora, and necklace pod saphora, as these may be the most poisonous plants in the cytisine class.

FRUIT SEEDS. Apple seeds are poisonous? Yes, it's true. However, it takes a substantial ingestion of well-chewed apple seeds to cause a poisoning. Apples and other fruit trees in the rose family—

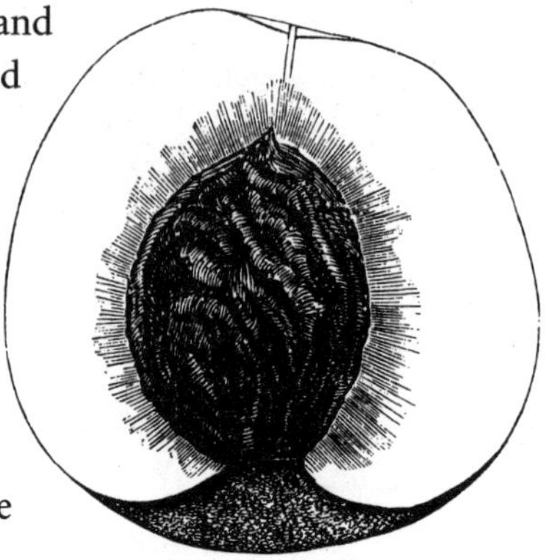

almonds, apricots, cherries, peaches, and plums—contain a compound called amygdalin, a relative of cyanide. While eating an entire apple, seeds and all, is not going to cause cyanide poisoning, there's some risk that consistently doing so can eventually result in a problem. Also, if for some strange reason you're into eating fruit tree bark, be aware that it also contains amygdalin.

AZALEAS AND RHODODENDRONS. Bees might look happy as they flit from azalea flower to rhododendron bloom, but actually they are slowly being poisoned. The same thing can happen to humans who eat parts of these popular bushes. Azaleas and rhododendrons contain grayanotoxins, poisons that cause gastrointestinal symptoms initially and later affect the blood pressure and heart.

Don't worry about a couple of azalea flowers or leaves. But if it's more than that, the ingestion is best handled in the emergency room. Other bushes that contain grayanotoxins include mountain laurel, sheep laurel, and dog laurel, also the ominously named lambkill and dogkill.

PYROLLIZIDINE ALKALOIDS. If you're into herbal medicine, you've surely heard of comfrey. Once popularly brewed as an herbal tea, comfrey has fallen from favor because it's been found to cause liver damage. Comfrey is one of the pyrollizidine plants, a group that also includes the popular annual dusty miller and the perennial genus *Heliotropium.*

Single ingestions of a pyrollizidine plant almost never cause poisoning. It's the long-term chronic exposures that do the damage. That's why grazing cattle are most susceptible to the pyrollizidine plants, many of which grow in the wild.

What about common yard weeds? Dandelions are not poisonous; in fact, some cultures use the leaves in salad and the flowers to make wine. Forget-me-nots and violets are nonpoisonous. Some types of clover are edible, but others contain chemicals that can irritate the stomach and interfere with normal blood clotting.

Killer Plants

Many plants have low-level toxicity; that is, you have to ingest a fairly substantial amount before symptoms occur. Not so with the killer plants. This group is so toxic that even small amounts—a leaf, a flower, a taste of sap—can result in a disaster.

OLEANDER. Let's put the toxicity of oleander in cow terms. A three-hundred-pound cow can die after eating just half a tablespoonful of an oleander plant. A single leaf can kill a human. Oleander contains the same kind of ingredients you'll find in the heart drug digoxin. On ingestion, this toxin causes the heart to beat in an irregular fashion, thereby driving down blood pressure. There may be severe gastrointestinal symptoms, like bloody diarrhea, before the respiratory system shuts down. *Everything about the oleander plant is poisonous.* That includes the water in which cut flowers of oleander might be kept and any smoke that results from burning the plant.

Other plants that similarly affect the heart include the Christmas rose, foxglove (digitalis), lily cf the valley, wild hyacinth, and squill.

CASTOR BEAN. Grown commercially for its laxative oil, the castor bean plant produces seeds that, when chewed, are deadly. Again, *they must be chewed to be toxic.* The seeds contain something called ricin, which is poisonous to intestinal cells, and ricinus agglutinin, a compound that breaks down red blood cells. Together, these two cause bloody diarrhea, ferocious cramps, and, eventually, liver and kidney failure.

Usually, there's a delayed reaction to the toxin. So even if nothing happens after a few hours or even days after the ingestion of castor seeds, it's imperative to seek medical treatment. It takes just one to three seeds to kill a child; two to six to kill an adult. The rosary pea may be even more toxic, with just one well-chewed seed capable of killing a child.

A few related plants that are not quite as toxic as these include the bellyache bush, black acacia, black locust, croton (technically not a member of the castor oil family, but a strong purgative nonetheless), and purge nut. As you can tell from the names, there's a common theme to these plants: Each causes intense intestinal irritation. In general, the safest bet is to avoid any inedible bean plant.

AUTUMN CROCUS. These are not the flowers that pop up out of the frozen earth in February but an autumn-blooming variety, also called meadow saffron, from which the drug colchicine is derived. Colchicine, used to treat gout, works much like an anticancer drug in that it inhibits normal cellular division. It tends to affect most those cells in the body that turn over rapidly: intestinal cells, cells in the bone marrow, and hair cells.

Colchicine is slowly absorbed. For perhaps twelve to even forty-eight hours following the ingestion of even a few seeds of the autumn crocus, nothing happens. Take advantage of this tremendous window of opportunity for treatment. Colchicine causes massive diarrhea that can lead to kidney damage and death. All parts of the autumn crocus are poisonous.

WATER HEMLOCK. This is not a plant you'll typically find growing around the yard, but you might encounter it in a moist area in the wild. The water hemlock is sometimes mistaken for such edible plants as the parsnip, which is a deadly mistake. Shortly after ingesting a bit of the root, severe gastrointestinal symptoms will ensue, followed by seizures, tremors, and paralysis of the respiratory muscles. Death can occur within an hour.

YEW. Used to make an anticancer drug, the yew tree has berries, inside of which are some extremely poisonous seeds. Chewing up even a small number of these seeds could result in an irregular heartbeat, leading to cardiac failure and death. If you have a yew tree in your yard, consider removing the berries from it. The leaves aren't as poisonous.

DEADLY NIGHTSHADE. Though it falls under the category of a solanine, deadly nightshade, or belladonna, is poisonous because of the scopolamine and hyoscyamine it contains. A child who ingests a few deadly nightshade berries will have typical "anticholinergic" symptoms: flushed skin, dry mouth, and a high fever.

JIMSONWEED AND MORNING GLORY. Those looking for a natural high will sometimes turn to jimsonweed, but it's a mistake. Certainly, a few leaves or seeds of jimsonweed may provide the desired delirium, but it comes at a cost: intense side effects that range from excessive fever to dangerous changes in blood pressure. Jimsonweed is a dangerous gamble. Stay away from it.

And if you think you're going to get high by eating morning glory seeds, think again. True, they contain a weak, LSD-like component. But the key here is *weak.* Tremendous numbers of seeds must be eaten, and many seeds these days are treated with noxious fungicides to discourage ingestion.

MUSHROOMS. The best rule: All wild mushrooms are toxic. While this may or may not be true, you need to be an expert to tell the difference between a safe and a poisonous mushroom. And even mushroom experts make mistakes—witness the "expert" foragers who cooked up some fungi in California in 1996, leaving one of those who ate the mushrooms, a young girl, needing a liver transplant.

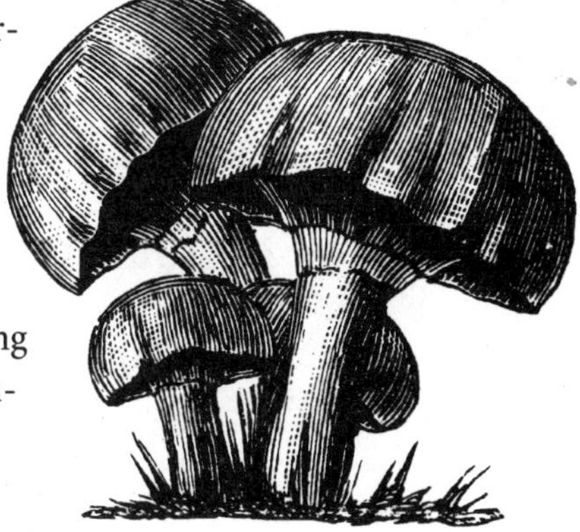

Poisonous mushrooms fall into two basic categories: ones that will affect you now, and ones that will affect you later. Within those categories is a wide range of toxins, producing many different effects. The "GI" mushrooms cause nothing more than nausea, vomiting, and diarrhea. "Muscarinic" mushrooms cause sweating and blurry vision. "Disulfiram" mushrooms cause no effects unless you take them with alcohol; then a list of highly unpleasant symptoms kicks in, from headache to nausea and vomiting. Some mushrooms can make you hallucinate ("muscimol" mushrooms), while others can produce liver damage (amanita mushrooms) or cause symptoms that mimic diabetes (cortinarius mushrooms).

But none of these specific effects really matter to a poison center. They can't identify mushrooms and don't even try. It's too risky. The safest method is to treat all mushroom ingestions as if they're potentially deadly. That means the use of ipecac syrup at home, if the ingestion has just occurred, or emergency room treatment if more than, say, thirty to sixty minutes has passed.

Then it's a matter of simple observation. If abdominal cramping, nausea, and vomiting occur within six to twelve hours, we know a highly toxic mushroom has been ingested, perhaps one from the deadly amanita family. *Get prompt medical attention if these symptoms occur, even if they seem to resolve on their own.* And these symptoms often *do* resolve on their own, giving the impression that the poisoning is over with. But it's not. One or two days later, the mushroom toxin begins killing liver cells. It also affects kidney function. In the end, a victim poisoned by an amanita mushroom faces permanent damage to the liver and possibly death.

Poison-proof Your Garden

Yes, you *can* have a beautiful and nontoxic garden. But a word of caution: *Know exactly what flower you have.* A rose may always be a rose, but many other common plant names are misused. For example, loosestrife to some means a tall plant with pink flowers,

It's a Fact

- Grass and grass seed are considered nontoxic.
- Cardinal flower plants are most poisonous just before and after they bloom.
- Green potatoes can be made safe again by storing in darkness for a few weeks. Once they have turned completely brown they are once again low enough in solanine to eat.
- Not all members of the lily family are poisonous. Take asparagus, for example, or chives, garlic, and leeks.
- Berries from plants in the solanine family, like the Jerusalem cherry, are more toxic when the berries are unripe.
- Boxwood is a toxic plant that is particularly attractive in floral arrangements. But florists generally use the nontoxic false boxwood in arrangements these days instead of the real thing.
- Think you have nothing in the house to treat poison ivy? Try rubbing on any aluminum-containing antiperspirant.
- Never burn poison ivy, oak, or sumac. Burning the plants releases extremely irritating fumes. Use a vine-killing chemical instead.
- Do not confuse the saffron crocus with the meadow saffron crocus. The former is the plant that gives us saffron, the expensive yellow herb; the latter is another name for the deadly colchicine-containing autumn crocus.
- The highly poisonous autumn crocus can be found for sale in bulb catalogs. If you have children in the house *don't buy it.* Spring-blooming varieties of crocus are far less toxic.

while others identify loosestrife as a bushy plant with drooping white flower heads. Always try to get a scientific name for the flower you want to identify; then call the poison center to check on its toxicity.

Here are some plants that generally won't cause any problem if ingested:

- Ageratum
- Asters (many)
- Astilbe
- Balloon flower
- Bee balm
- Cosmos
- Ferns (most varieties)
- Forget-me-nots (true perennial)
- Gayfeather
- Gomphrena
- Honeysuckle
- Impatiens
- Jacob's ladder
- Johnny jump-up (viola)
- Monkey grass (liriope)
- Nandina
- Nasturtium
- Pansy
- Phlox
- Plumbago
- Portulaca
- Pot marigolds
- Rose campion
- Sweet alyssum
- Zinnia

Other Yard Hazards

Swimming Pool Products

Be extremely careful not to inhale swimming pool chlorine. It's highly concentrated and will cause severe coughing, wheezing, problems breathing, and perhaps the development of pneumonia with even short periods of exposure.

If it does happen, immediately get fresh air. Coughing should subside over a period of about thirty minutes, but if it doesn't, or if wheezing is severe, call 911. If you recover from the initial symptoms only to develop the same ones later on, go to the emergency room. It could indicate pneumonia has developed.

Swimming pool chlorine is equally dangerous to the eyes. Begin rinsing them out immediately with lukewarm water and don't stop until thirty minutes has gone by. In the meantime, have someone make arrangements to get you to a hospital.

Never allow children to disinfect the swimming pool or help "shock" it in the fall.

If your pool filter uses diatomaceous earth, by the way, it's non-toxic.

The Grill

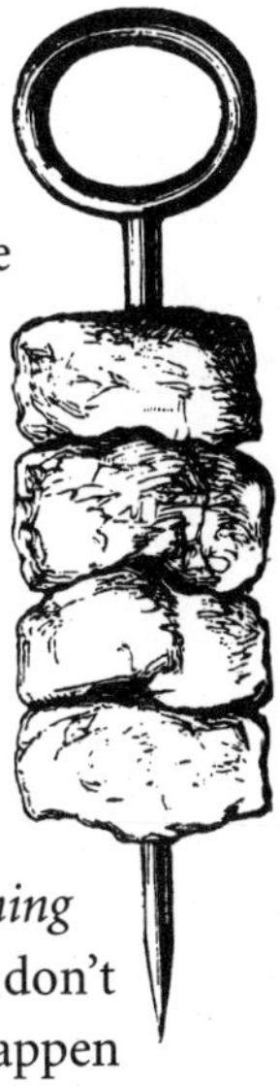

In the short run, the most toxic grill product is lighter fluid. (Long-term, it's the carcinogens in the grilled food.) Charcoal starters contain petroleum products that, when swallowed, can drip into the lungs. This sets the stage for chemical pneumonitis, a potentially deadly condition in which the lungs become inflamed and fill up with fluid.

Treatment

Here's what to do for a mouthful of lighter fluid. First, *do not induce vomiting.* The last thing we want is to give the lighter fluid a second opportunity to find its way into the lungs. Second, *give little or nothing by mouth for two hours* following an exposure. We don't want to stimulate vomiting, and that's what might happen if you start forcing fluid down the throat. Instead, sips of water, milk, or juice will do for the first two hours. After that, observe for four more hours. If any "chest-cold" symptoms develop during that time—coughing, wheezing, fever, complaints of pain on breathing in—go to the emergency room. If not, you're home free.

Lighter fluid has a strong smell, and those who ingest it will complain even up to a day later that they can smell and taste it. There is nothing you can do about this. If the lighter fluid causes an upset stomach, use an antacid.

Charcoal itself is nontoxic, ditto for charcoal ashes. However, a big chunk of anything can cause choking.

Around the House

Concrete and Mortar

Patching up the sidewalk? Wear gloves and boots, if you're using concrete or cement. These products are corrosive and can burn and blister exposed skin. Seek medical help if you sustain a concrete burn, as tissue damage can be severe. Mortar is slightly less corrosive but is still a strong irritant.

3

The Kitchen

Fortunately, most poisonous items found in the kitchen tend to be of lower toxicity than those elsewhere in the house, for the simple reason that they are used around food.

Cleaning Products

Soaps to Wash the Dishes

Here's a fact you need to know: The soap you put in the dishwasher is far more toxic than what you use in the sink. Dishwasher soap has a rather high pH. A product's pH measures its potential to damage tissue. An extremely high pH—up around 12 or 13—is especially dangerous, as is an extremely low pH—anything below, say, 3. For a reference point, keep in mind that the pH of most bodily fluids is around 7.

Most machine dishwasher soaps have pHs above 10 because they contain the corrosive products sodium carbonate and sodium silicate. Hand dishwashing soaps, which do not have these chemicals, have a pH closer to 7. However, not every dishwasher product is corrosive. Some are worse than others. Check with your poison center about the danger of your favorite brand.

Treatment

As far as poisonings go, these differences in pH mean little unless you have one of those products up in the 12 or 13 range. Then, actual burns are possible. Treatment for an ingestion of either hand or machine dish soap is the same at first: Rinse out the mouth completely and give a small glass of water, juice, or milk. Expect vomiting to occur. Once the vomiting clears, there should be few, if any, residual symptoms. If, however, you notice burns or blisters inside the mouth or on the lips, excessive drooling, or complaints that swallowing hurts, go to the emergency room.

A splash of any type of soap into the eyes will *feel* corrosive, pH figures notwithstanding. But most eye exposures to dish soaps—hand or machine—can be treated at home with a fifteen-minute lukewarm-water eye wash. Once the rinsing is finished, allow about a forty-five-minute cool-down period, then reexamine the eyes. If they still look red, swollen, and teary, see a doctor. With the higher pH dishwasher soaps, do an extra ten to fifteen minutes of rinsing and plan to see a doctor when you're through.

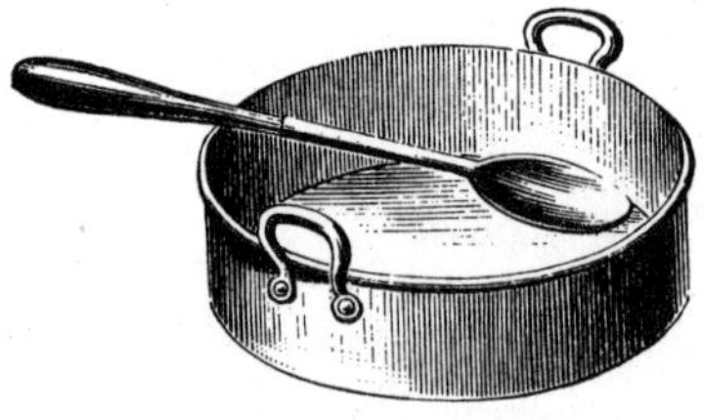

Cleansers

Sink cleansers—powder or liquid—are chemically quite similar to hand dishwashing soaps. So an ingested cleanser should cause nothing more than mild vomiting, and in the eyes, redness and slight swelling. Give a glass of water, juice, or milk for a cleanser ingestion; for the eyes, rinse for fifteen minutes with lukewarm water. Medical treatment isn't usually necessary for cleanser exposures. Treat ingestions of rinsing agents—those little basketfuls you put in the dishwasher (Jet Dry, for example)—the same way.

Soap Pads

The ubiquitous Brillo and S.O.S. pads are really just steel wool embedded with soap. While it's hard to imagine anyone chomping on a Brillo pad, anything is possible. The soap might cause mild vomiting. The pad itself would be treated as a "foreign body" ingestion—meaning that it's not poisonous, but that some pieces, if big enough, could cause abrasions in the throat, stomach, or intestines. Look for blood in the vomitus or complaints of stomach or throat pain after the vomiting has resolved. Go to the emergency room if these occur.

Window Washers

Window cleaners come in such a pretty shade of blue it's no wonder children often take a swallow. The good news about commercial window cleaners is that they're very low in toxicity because you're mostly buying water. Sure, there are some with a bit of ammonia and vinegar, and most contain a splash of a very toxic solvent called ethylene glycol butyl ether. But the solutions are so dilute there's very little chance of a poisoning. Give a glass of water, juice, or milk. In the eyes, a simple fifteen-minute rinse will suffice.

Floor Polishes

Acrylic floor waxes contain a bit more of ethylene glycol butyl ether, that toxic solvent, but it's still almost unheard-of to see symptoms after a small exposure—a swallow, for example. Once again, give a glass of fluid and observe for mild vomiting.

Household Ammonia

Want to see a distressing sight? Watch someone take a swallow of household ammonia. The pungent, overpowering smell causes gagging, coughing, vomiting, and tearing of the eyes. There may even be swelling around the mouth. But despite the theatrics, household ammonia is actually low in toxicity. It's the concentrated industrial ammonia that can kill.

When swallowed, household ammonia irritates the mouth and throat, often stimulating the gag reflex and subsequent vomiting. Large ingestions of ammonia—such as might occur in a suicide attempt—can burn the throat.

To treat ammonia ingestions first get fresh air. Next, take sips of water, milk, or juice. That should do it. The fluid may stimulate vomiting, but whether it does or not is of little consequence. If, hours later, burning sensations develop in the throat or there's trouble swallowing or excessive drooling, see a doctor.

Ammonia is *extremely* irritating to the eyes. Splash lukewarm water into the eyes for about twenty minutes following an ammonia exposure, then let the eyes cool down for about forty minutes before checking them again for excessive irritation. Use your judgment. If they still look or feel bad, go to the emergency room. Skin exposures tend to be mild. Wash thoroughly with soap and water.

Ammonia smells like the extract of a thousand bad onions, and excessive inhalation of its noxious fumes can inflame the lungs. If fresh air doesn't relieve the coughing and wheezing, or the symptoms return hours later, see a doctor.

It's a Fact

- Pneumonia from ammonia? Mixing ammonia with bleach produces a deadly gas called chloramine. In a high concentration, chloramine causes chemical pneumonitis, a severe inflammation of the lungs. *Never mix ammonia with bleach or any other household cleaning agent.*
- What was once the source of ammonia for Britain's dye industry? Human urine.
- Another synonym for ammonia is spirits of hartshorn, because it was once made from the hoofs and horns of oxen.
- Smelling salts have an ammonia base.

Pine Oil Cleaners

For the most part, a swallow of a pine oil cleaner—the most anyone can usually stand—will not cause serious symptoms. Pine oil is a rubefacient—a substance that causes redness and irritation, the very symptoms you'll see around the lips, the mouth, and in the throat. But two possible problems complicate pine oil ingestions. First, pine oil can be aspirated into the lungs. That can set up chemical pneumonia. Second, pine oil itself, if taken in a sufficient quantity—and we'd be talking here about a chug-a-lug on the pine cleaner bottle—causes drowsiness and even coma.

Put all that together and we come up with two very important words when it comes to pine oil cleaners: no ipecac. We don't want to irritate the throat and mouth again, expose the lungs a second time to an oily substance, or have a patient vomiting while drowsy.

Instead, clean out the mouth with a soft wet cloth and encourage sips—only sips—of water or juice. Don't overload the stomach with fluid or it might stimulate vomiting. Look for drowsiness, in the first ninety minutes after the exposure, and for respiratory symptoms for four to six hours after. You're home free if neither occurs by then. For a large exposure go directly to the emergency room.

Pine oil, by its oily nature, creates a sustained period of irritation in the eyes that may require up to thirty minutes of lukewarm-water rinsing to relieve. Usually, no follow-up medical treatment is needed.

Oven Cleaners

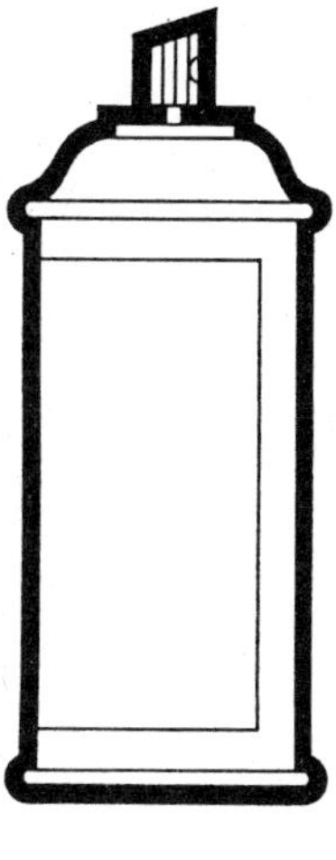

Cleaning the oven: worst job, worst poison. Remember that mini-course on pH a few poisons back? It becomes especially important when you're dealing with oven cleaners. By and large, these products are corrosive, with pH values near or higher than 13. They are extremely dangerous to eat, splash in the eyes, or get on the skin.

Around the House

First, a bit of obvious preventive advice: Always wear rubber gloves when using an oven cleaner. Alkaline burns tend to come on slowly. Without gloves, by the time you realize you've been burned, a minor medical situation might have turned into something major. If you do splash oven cleaner on the skin, wash it off thoroughly with warm water and soap. Some irritation will linger. If you notice any blistering or a loss of sensation in the burn area, see a doctor.

Most oven cleaners come as sprays, and that puts the eyes at risk for an exposure. *Spraying oven cleaner into the eyes is a medical emergency.* Immediately begin rinsing the eyes with lukewarm water and continue doing so for thirty minutes. During that time, have someone arrange hospital transportation, as the eyes need to be examined for burns.

Ingesting an oven cleaner can also be a medical emergency—depending on the amount. A family member, unaware the oven is being cleaned, might pop something in, heat it up, and eat it. Usually, this type of an exposure is not a big deal. You could watch for signs of throat damage—a change in the way the voice sounds, drooling instead of swallowing, difficulty swallowing—but they're not likely to occur. For ingestion of a large or unknown amount of oven cleaner, go immediately to the emergency room. *Do not under any circumstances use ipecac syrup after the ingestion of a corrosive oven cleaner.*

Foods

Salt

Numerous home remedies exist to stimulate vomiting, and all of them are dangerous. There's the stick the finger down the throat method (which can damage tissues there) and the raw egg method (which can give you food poisoning). But perhaps the most dangerous home emetic is heavily salted water.

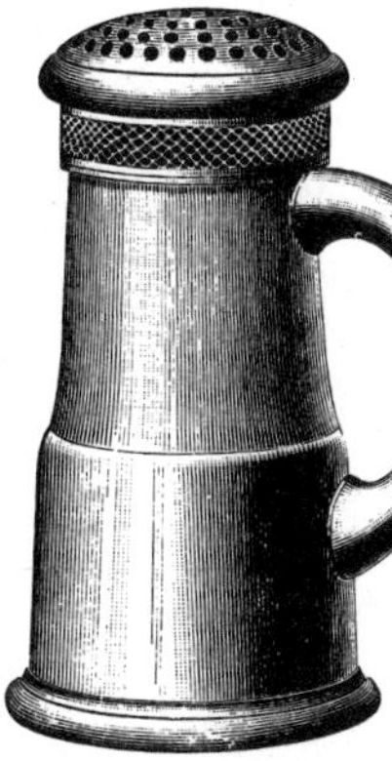

Salt, that most common of condiments, is poisonous. And while no one is likely to sit down with a container of Morton's and a spoon, the saltwater-vomiting treatment sometimes exposes children to toxic amounts of sodium chloride. How much salt will cause poisoning? In general, for every twelve pounds of body weight, ingesting half a teaspoonful of salt could edge the body's delicate balance of sodium and chloride into a dangerous range.

Go easy on the salt. Where salt goes, water follows. And in the body, an excess of salt causes a drain of water from the cells. Eventually, the cells become so dehydrated they die. That's why those with salt poisoning will seem lethargic—some of their brain cells are dead or dying.

Let the emergency room handle salt poisonings. Electrolytes need to be monitored and IV fluids given.

Sodium Bicarbonate

Like salt, sodium bicarbonate gets absorbed and can potentially affect the body's electrolyte balance. So never use baking soda or baking powder as an antacid unless specifically instructed to do so by a doctor. Single small ingestions of baking soda are generally not a problem. But chronic use of pure baking soda for an upset stomach can affect virtually every organ system in the body.

Mold

Food molds are a bit like mushrooms: You never know when you might get one that's extremely toxic. While in the past it was thought that cutting out moldy spots on food made them acceptable to eat, that's no longer the case. While many food molds might cause nothing more than mild nausea, vomiting, or diarrhea, some are highly toxic. Plus, mold toxins sink down into the food past the area of apparent mold colonization. So cutting out the mold may not remove all the poison. The safest thing to do with a moldy piece of food is to throw it out.

It's a Fact

• Got a family member who's allergic to penicillin? Keep them away from food molds, some of which can contain the antibiotic.

• One of the most infamous (and deadly) food mold problems is the ergot contamination of grain. The ergot alkaloids cause intense constriction of blood vessels, in some cases leading to the loss of outlying body parts like fingers. Fortunately, where the U.S. food supply is concerned, ergot contamination is mostly of historical interest.

• Another highly toxic mold occurs on peanuts and corn. Ingesting aflatoxin may cause cancer in the long run. Remember, food molds found in peanut butter and cereal grains may be highly dangerous.

Silver Cake Balls

Yes, they contain silver. But toxicity from eating silver cake balls is almost unheard-of. Enjoy—in moderation. And taking a nibble from a birthday candle isn't a problem either. Candles are nontoxic.

Jalapeño Peppers

Okay, all you salsa makers out there. What's the most important ingredient you need when preparing a fresh batch of dip? The answer isn't tomatoes, cilantro, or even peppers—it's gloves. That's because the jalapeño peppers you need for salsa can burn your fingers. Not actual burns, of course, but intense irritation that lasts and lasts.

Unfortunately, there's no definitive cure for jalapeño hands—only a bunch of home remedies with a spotty record of success. Lets go over them.

First, of course, you'll want to wash thoroughly with soap and water. Next, some people advocate soaking the hands in cold water. Others suggest warm water. Water doesn't work, others say;

it's vegetable oil that does the trick. There are still two more camps: one suggests a soak in milk; another, vinegar.

It's likely you'll try every one of these methods and still not find perfect relief. Jalapeño hands are one of the most stubborn things to get rid of. If these home remedies fail you, trot down to the pharmacy and ask for some Xylocaine jelly. It's a little expensive, but when you slather it on, you might find the relief worth the money.

Oh, one more home remedy, recommended by a chef: Smear toothpaste over the affected area.

Fumes

Putting Out Fires

Ever wonder what's inside those mini fire extinguishers used to squelch the occasional stovetop blaze? Well, you need to know. Because in the literal heat of the moment, fire extinguishers get sprayed haphazardly, and it isn't unusual to take an extinguisher blast in the face.

Most home extinguishers contain either sodium bicarbonate or ammonium phosphate, both of which irritate the eyes. The ammonium phosphate also irritates the skin, and both products, given their particulate nature, cause coughing and a scratchy throat if inhaled.

> **It's a Fact**
>
> • Some foam fire extinguishers may contain highly poisonous ethylene glycol.
>
> • Other nontoxic ingredients found in fire extinguishers include boric acid, graphite, and clay particles.

Are any of these effects dangerous? Probably not. Those with asthma are at higher risk of respiratory difficulties if exposed to fire extinguisher fumes, and nearly everyone exposed will need to seek fresh air and perhaps rinse out the eyes for ten to fifteen minutes with lukewarm water. Any persistent eye irritation, wheezing, or coughing should be treated by a doctor.

Freon

Occasionally, refrigerators will leak freon. Is freon dangerous? Yes. Do refrigerators (and air conditioners) contain enough freon to be hazardous if a leak occurs? Probably not.

Freon has two main effects on the body. First, it's irritating to the eyes and respiratory system, but minor coughing, sneezing, and stinging of the eyes is usually all you'll see with a home freon leak. But freon has an additional, more serious effect on the heart: It sensitizes cardiac tissue into producing erratic heartbeats.

Again, it's highly unlikely such a reaction would occur from a home freon leak. But take precautions anyway. Open all the windows in the kitchen and get outside into fresh air. If the freon leak has occurred late in the day and you can't get the appliance fixed until morning, it's safe to stay in the house provided you keep the kitchen windows open.

It's a Fact

• When burned, freon releases highly poisonous gases such as phosgene. So during a freon leak, be sure the kitchen is well ventilated before you light up the stove.

• How do you know if you've got a freon leak? First, you might hear a soft hiss coming from the appliance as the gas passes through a hole; second, the room may smell like a freshly cut lawn.

• The ozone layer is highly susceptible to destruction by freon, and it's freon's chlorine molecule that does the damage. One chlorine atom can destroy up to one hundred thousand atoms of ozone.

• How's this for environmental notoriety? The same man credited with discovering the refrigerant properties of freon is also the man who suggested adding lead to gasoline to prevent knocking.

Teflon

Teflon was discovered in 1938 when DuPont chemist Roy J. Plunkett found a solid, deflective material inside a cylinder that was supposed to contain a gas.

Teflon, completely nontoxic as

a solid, forms irritating toxic gases when it's burned. But you have to burn it at an extremely high temperature to get those gases, one that's usually unattainable in the average kitchen. Perhaps you've got one of those super BTU stoves. If so, and you burn a Teflon pan, open all the windows and leave the room. Once the room is aired out, you should have no further problem.

Freezer Packs

They're meant to be used *for* injuries, but if the liquid in a reusable ice pack is ingested, it could cause an injury: methemoglobinemia, a blood condition associated with the ingestion of nitrates—ammonium nitrate, in the case of ice packs. But unless someone sucks on an ice pack and swallows a substantial amount of the fluid inside, there won't be a problem.

And those sealed reusable ice cubes? They're nontoxic.

Food Poisoning

You know that little "stomach virus" you got last month, that touch of diarrhea, that spell of vomiting? Odds are it could've been food poisoning.

Every so often, you'll find food poisoning in the news, usually after some catastrophe. How many of us remember the Bon Vivant vichyssoise soup scare of the 1970s? A batch of that canned potato soup, traditionally served cold, was apparently contaminated with botulism toxin.

Food poisoning is a ubiquitous but mostly hidden disorder—one that comes and goes in the space of a day or two, leaving behind only unpleasant memories of many trips to the bathroom. By far, most cases of food poisoning resolve on their own in twenty-four to forty-eight hours and can be treated at home by giving fluids.

Before embarking on fluid therapy, however, make sure you've got food poisoning and not some acute emergency like appendicitis or a kidney stone. The symptoms of gastroenteritis—the stomach kind of food poisoning—are simple: abdominal cramps and diarrhea. Sometimes nausea and vomiting may develop, as well, and a light fever is possible.

Treatment

To some extent, it hardly matters what organism is causing the intestinal symptoms. The treatment is the same in every case: Prevent dehydration by giving plenty of clear fluids. If at any point you've got a food poisoning victim too weak to drink fluids, or one who's also vomiting and can't hold liquid down, you have an emergency that needs to be treated in the hospital.

Other exceptions to the treat-at-home rule:

1. When a child or elderly person is involved. Diarrhea is especially dangerous in infants and toddlers because it dehydrates them quickly. Elderly people have the same problem. *Seek medical help for any sustained bout of diarrhea in a small child or an elderly person.*

2. When there's blood in the diarrhea in a person of any age. It could indicate poisoning by salmonella, shigella, or a deadly strain of *Escherichia coli.*

Escherichia coli

The last time food poisoning made headlines, we learned there was a new and deadly strain of *E. coli* out there named 0157:H7. A harmless strain of *E. coli* exists in the human intestinal tract, so where did this killer come from? It's possible it could have mutated in response to antibiotics fed to cattle, but no one is really sure. Or unsanitary conditions in the meat-processing plant might have allowed infected cattle feces to get mixed in with ground beef, and *E. coli* 0157:H7 to enter the food chain; no one is sure about that either. In fact, we're not even sure eating meat is the only way to get infected with 0157:H7. A huge outbreak of 0157:H7 poisoning in Japan was tentatively traced to radish sprouts.

We *are* sure of one thing: *E. coli* 0157:H7 infections can be deadly. Several died after eating undercooked hamburgers infected with the bacterium in what became known as the Jack-in-the-Box incident, so named because that's where some of the poisonous hamburgers were purchased.

The toxin from *E. coli* 0157:H7 causes not just diarrhea but *bloody* diarrhea, which can lead to something called hemolytic uremic syndrome—basically, kidney failure secondary to the destruction of blood cells.

While new food inspection rules may solve the problem of 0157:H7 outbreaks, consumers can protect themselves by making sure all ground meat dishes are *cooked thoroughly.* That means *no pink and no blood in the juices.* All juices running from the meat should be clear. If you see any blood, you have not cooked the meat enough. You might also consider forgoing the feeding of ground meat products to small children.

To reiterate: *The presence of bloody diarrhea may indicate a severe form of food poisoning and should always be treated by a doctor.*

Salmonella

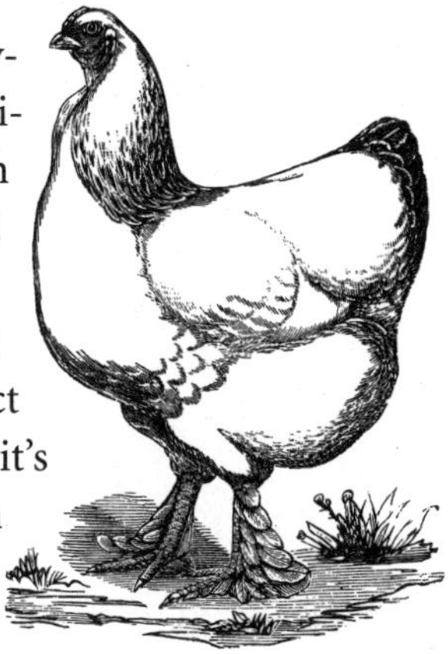

You had breakfast a few days ago—eggs, sunny-side up—and this morning you woke with terrible cramps, diarrhea, and chills alternating with fever. The diagnosis: probably salmonella food poisoning.

The first clue: eggs or chicken that weren't thoroughly cooked. While salmonella can infect almost any food—even the surface of fruits—it's most commonly linked in the United States with poultry products. The second clue: the delay between eating the infected food and developing the symptoms. With other "stomach" food poisonings, symptoms usually hit soon after ingesting the bad food, and the entire illness resolves in a day or two. But salmonella bacteria need a couple of days just to multiply in the intestinal tract.

Salmonella infections can be more severe than other food poisonings, but if you're reasonably healthy even salmonellosis can be treated at home by giving lots of clear fluid. Once again, if the food poisoning victim is very young, very old, or sick in the first place with something else, they belong in the hospital with a salmonella infection. Bloody diarrhea can also occur with salmonellosis, though it's usually nowhere near as profuse as with *E. coli* 0157:H7.

How to Prevent Food Poisoning

Many cases of food poisoning could be prevented if cooks remembered one simple rule: Bacteria love warm, wet places, so avoid serving "warm" food. If something is supposed to be served hot, make sure it stays hot. If it's supposed to be cold, keep it cold.

Never prestuff a turkey. It's cozy and warm inside the belly of that bird. Instead, cook the stuffing separately in a dish.

Don't leave meat on the counter to thaw. Instead, keep it refrigerated during thawing. Never "slow-cook" meat in a warm oven. The minimum temperature for roasting meat is 325 degrees Fahrenheit. And never put cooked meat on the same plate that formerly held raw meat.

Cook food thoroughly. No runny eggs, no rare burgers.

Wash, wash, wash. Soap, water, and bleach are your best friends in the kitchen. When moving from food to food, wash with soap and water. When using a cutting board to prepare meat for cooking, wash the board with soap and water, then rinse it down with laundry bleach. When food preparation is finished, wipe the counters down with soap and water, then bleach. Bleach is an excellent disinfectant. Use it.

It's a Fact

• Salmonella was named for Daniel Elmer Salmon, an accomplished veterinarian.

• You cannot contract salmonella through an open cut. You can, however, infect meat via an open cut.

• More than half of all food poisonings may be caused by salmonella.

• Despite their virulence when ingested, salmonella bacteria are easily killed by five minutes of boiling.

• A salmonella infection can sometimes be confused with one caused by shigella, named for Kiyoshi Shiga. Shigellosis more frequently causes bloody diarrhea.

• Because poultry is often sold with the skin still attached to the meat, it carries a higher risk of bacterial contamination. Skin has a higher bacteria count than flesh.

• "Buffet table" food poisoning is often caused by *Staphylococcus aureus.* The hallmark of a staph food poisoning is the quick onset of cramping and diarrhea. Reheating food that's been left out on a counter won't necessarily stop a staph food poisoning. That's because the toxin secreted by staph bacteria isn't destroyed by heat.

• *Listeria* infections (named for surgeon Joseph Lister) are usually associated with unpasteurized dairy products and can be deadly. In 1987, more than sixty died in California after ingesting Listeria-tainted cheese.

• Lysozyme, an enzyme found in human tears that protects the eye from infection, is lethal to *Listeria* bacteria.

• Pregnant women should *never* eat unpasteurized dairy products, because *Listeria* is especially toxic to the developing fetus.

• The so-called twenty-four-hour bug is commonly caused by *Clostridium perfringens,* a bacterium that contaminates meat and fish.

Don't refreeze thawed-out meat. Not only does refreezing destroy the texture of the meat, but toxins may also have formed during thawing.

Don't sample cake batters that contain raw eggs, and discard eggs with cracks or visible dirt.

Botulism

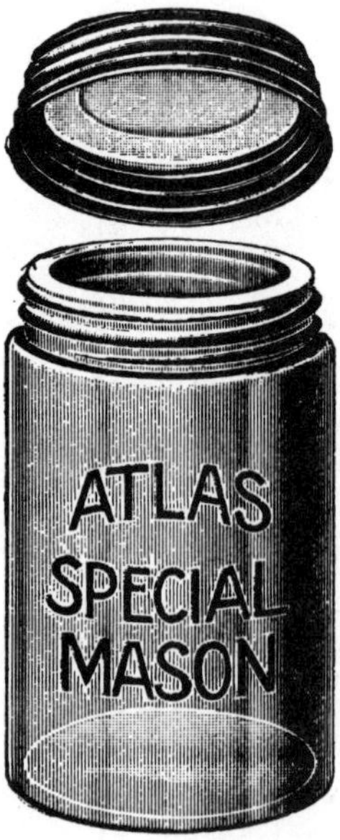

Now back to the case of the Bon Vivant vichyssoise soup that caused a couple of cases of botulism poisoning back in 1971. There are several clues in that poisoning that tell us much of what we need to know about botulism. First, by and large botulism occurs in canned foods. That's got nothing to do with the can but with the lack of oxygen. Botulism spores cannot survive in an oxygen-rich environment. Second, the soup was served cold. While botulism spores are highly resistant to heat, botulism toxin—the stuff that causes the problems—is easily destroyed by about ten minutes of boiling. And, finally, potato soup is likely a low-acid food. Acidic environments hinder the development of botulism.

What is botulism? It's an unusual—and fortunately very rare—form of food poisoning that affects the nervous system. At its worst, botulism causes paralysis of the respiratory muscles and death. Botulism rarely occurs with commercially canned products; it is more common with home-canned goods. Ideally, you should do no home canning. But if you insist, make sure everything used in the process is clean, sterile, and heated past the boiling point.

Food spoiled with botulism may look and smell foul or it may not. So follow a simple rule with canned foods: *When in doubt, throw it out.* One almost sure sign of botulism is a can that's swollen or that propels food when opened. That's because the botulism spores produce gas. Dented cans, on the other hand, are not necessarily suspect.

If you think you may have eaten something contaminated with botulism, call your local poison center. Most times, you'll be instructed to watch for symptoms, which usually take fifteen to twenty-four hours to develop—sometimes longer. A sore throat

It's a Fact

• Botulism toxin is so poisonous that it would take no more than seven ounces to kill every human being on the planet.

• The word "botulism" is derived from the Latin word for sausage, as the first outbreaks of botulism poisoning occurred in spoiled sausage.

• If there's any one home-canned food you should avoid it's mushrooms. Botulism spores are found in the soil, and mushrooms are difficult to get completely clean.

• Never prepare oil and garlic mixtures unless you plan to use them up quickly. By immersing garlic in oil you create an airless atmosphere in which botulism spores on the garlic could begin to release toxin. Commercial garlic-and-oil mixtures contain citric acid to retard this growth.

• The leading place you'll find botulism poisoning in the United States is in Alaska, where much of the food—especially meat—is preserved in ways that lock out oxygen. For example, some meats are immersed in oil, others encased in sealskin. Other "high botulism" states include Washington, Oregon, California, and Colorado.

• Honey has become a forbidden food for infants because it may transmit botulism bacteria that later grow in the intestinal tract and cause death. However, honey is probably not the only food to transmit "infant botulism."

and trouble focusing are early signs of botulism toxicity; weakness in the muscles, constipation, and fatigue may follow. Botulism poisonings must be treated with an antitoxin, so if these symptoms develop go right to the emergency room.

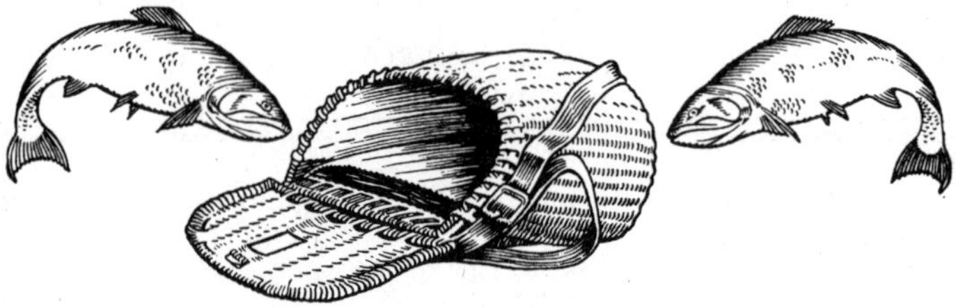

Scombroid Poisoning

Let's say you cook a piece of fish and find it tastes a bit peppery. Should you add a little salt and finish eating the fish or throw it away? The answer: Toss it. The peppery-tasting fish might cause a dramatic though generally harmless form of food poisoning known as scombroid poisoning. What's dramatic is how fast the poisoning comes on and how visible the symptoms: a vibrant red rash, sometimes accompanied by headache, dizziness, and gastrointestinal symptoms. The pepper taste of the fish indicates it contains high levels of histamine, the same chemical in humans that is secreted during an allergic reaction.

Many types of fish spoil without turning into slabs of histamine, so scombroid poisoning is rare. And it's usually a minor disorder that clears up quickly with the help of antihistamines. Still, it's such a distressing reaction that it's best handled in the emergency room.

It's a Fact

• Histamine can stand high temperatures for much longer periods of time than it takes to cook a piece of fish. So you can't cook scombroid poisoning out.

Shellfish Poisonings

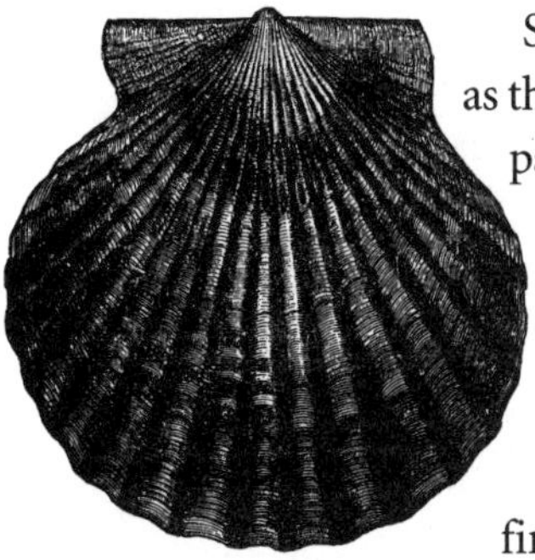

Shellfish don't become spoiled as much as they become contaminated. For example, paralytic shellfish poisoning occurs when shellfish feast on toxic microorganisms and then, in turn, are eaten by human beings. Neurotoxic shellfish poisoning occurs after the shellfish have been contaminated with ciguatera toxin. And finally, oysters in polluted waters sometimes become contaminated with *Vibrio vulnificus*, a relative of the organism that causes cholera. Compounding the problem is that oysters and some other shellfish are traditionally served raw.

Each of these food poisonings can result in death. So take no chances with shellfish. If they've been pulled from unapproved waters, steer clear of them.

It's a Fact

- Ciguatera toxin cannot be cooked out of shellfish.
- Shellfish—particularly oysters—should never be caught or eaten raw during the warm months, as they're more likely to be contaminated.
- Despite the bonhomie, oyster bars, where shellfish are consumed raw, are breeding grounds for serious illness and should be avoided. If you really want to enjoy a safe meal of oysters, cook them.

4

The Garage

Almost every poisonous material found in the garage is in the service of one thing: maintaining the family car. And most of these toxic products are derived from petroleum. That's actually good news, for with petroleum products there is a potential for toxicity that often doesn't materialize. And frankly, it's the nonpetroleum products in the garage that are most troublesome.

Antifreeze

By far the most poisonous things you'll find in the average garage are antifreezes made from methanol or ethylene glycol. Methanol is often found in windshield washer fluid, while ethylene glycol is used in the car's coolant system.

Methanol

Methanol, also called wood alcohol, was made famous earlier in this century when it was used by bootleggers during Prohibition to make alcoholic beverages. There was one catch with this ethanol substitute, however: Methanol causes blindness.

The body metabolizes methanol the same way it does an alcoholic beverage. But with methanol, a couple of toxic by-products are formed: formaldehyde and formic acid. The formic acid poisons eye tissue; the formaldehyde poisons everything else. These metabolites are killers because they make the blood more acidic, which upsets the delicate chemical balance that keeps our bodies running.

Remember, *any methanol ingestion is potentially dangerous.* Even as little as a teaspoonful has caused blindness, and hospital treatment is almost always necessary.

With the fatal attraction methanol has for eye tissue, you'd think a splash of windshield wiper fluid in the eyes would constitute a major problem. But remember, it's not the methanol itself that causes blindness, it's formic acid, a metabolite. Methanol irritates the eyes but doesn't harm them. So simply rinse out the eyes for ten to fifteen minutes with lukewarm water and see a doctor if irritation persists past an hour.

Methanol is not particularly toxic to the skin either. But, it can be *absorbed* through the skin. Never continue to wear methanol-soaked clothes. Immediately and thoroughly wash the skin.

Ethylene Glycol

The body also breaks ethylene glycol down into a set of toxic acids: glycolic acid, glyoxylic acid, and, finally, oxalic acid. Once again, we are dealing with acidic compounds that interfere with the body's normal functioning. But ethylene glycol also directly damages the kidneys, as sharp crystals of oxalic acid push their way through those organs on their way to the bladder.

As with methanol, *any ethylene glycol ingestion is potentially dangerous.* In most cases, poison centers will recommend an emergency room visit for antifreeze ingestions, even if they are small.

Brake Fluids

Brake fluids fall into the same category as radiator antifreeze: Most contain some sort of highly toxic glycol compound, usually diethylene glycol. How much brake fluid is toxic? It's hard to say. Manufacturers of automobile products tend to be secretive about their formulations, so sometimes we don't know how much glycol a particular brake fluid contains.

The best bet is to treat all brake fluid ingestions as potentially

It's a Fact

• One effective way to treat a methanol or ethylene glycol ingestion is by metabolic interference using ethanol—the kind of alcohol found in wine, beer, and spirits. Ethanol competes with methanol and ethylene glycol for the same enzyme and thus blocks transformation of these compounds into toxic metabolites.

• Be especially careful to wipe up any ethylene glycol antifreeze that might spill in the garage. Dogs and cats like the taste of ethylene glycol and can easily die from licking it off the floor.

• One early sign of intoxication with either methanol or ethylene glycol is uncoordination and symptoms of drunkeness. However, with methanol, those symptoms can take several hours to develop.

• Never pour ethylene glycol antifreeze into a hot radiator. It might vaporize in your face, and ethylene glycol is toxic when inhaled.

• Nonpoisonous antifreezes on the market usually contain propylene glycol. Propylene glycol is, in fact, low in toxicity.

toxic. Don't use ipecac syrup, as glycols can cause drowsiness. Instead, call the poison center and prepare to go to the emergency room.

Car Cleaning Products

Chrome Wheel Cleaners

In the 1800s, chemists faced a tough task: how to isolate fluorine. The problem was, fluorine formed an acid that was so strong it melted laboratory glassware. That acid—hydrofluoric—is one

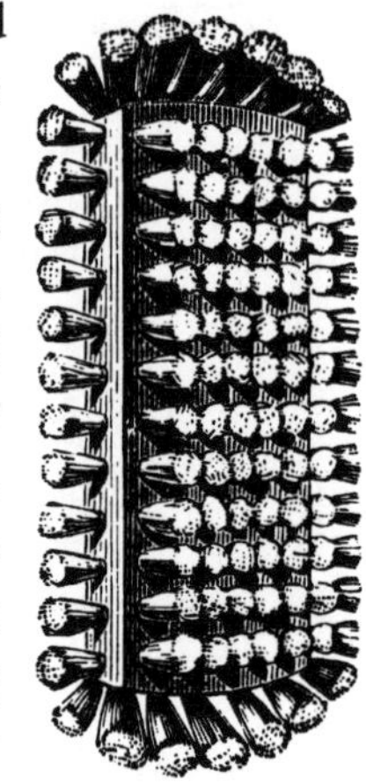

of the most dangerous products you'll find used in the home, most often as an ingredient in wire wheel cleaners.

Hydrofluoric acid not only burns the skin, it also binds to and depletes the mineral calcium. The heart and other muscles in the body depend on calcium to function properly. Thus, a big hydrofluoric acid burn could lead to a heart attack.

At home, most hydrofluoric acid burns are minor by comparison. But that doesn't mean they don't hurt, and it doesn't mean cleaning wire wheels isn't a dangerous task. It should only be done with gloves and eye protection and with adequate ventilation.

Hydrofluoric acid burns may go unnoticed at first. But within a few hours the area will begin to throb. The pain can become excrutiating and may indicate the tissues are severely damaged. *It is imperative that treatment for a hydrofluoric acid burn be supervised by medical personnel.*

That treatment could range from a home soak in Epsom salts—which contain magnesium, a molecule similar to calcium—to a hospital visit for treatment with calcium gluconate gel or calcium injections. Calcium and related molecules ease the pain from hydrofluoric acid burns by binding with and inactivating the fluoride.

As you can imagine, a spray of hydrofluoric acid to the eyes—even in the low concentrations found in most wire wheel cleaners—is an emergency. Immediately begin flushing the eyes with lukewarm water and continue doing so for up to thirty minutes. Then head to the emergency room. It's important to check for burns.

And finally, always use these wheel cleaners in fresh air. Inhaling hydrofluoric acid irritates the lungs, and chemical pneumonitis could develop.

Tire Cleaners

Putting hydrofluoric acid on a tire would probably melt the rubber, so most tire cleaners contain a nontoxic silicone compound. The silicone alone is not a big problem, but some of these products may also contain irritating soaps and waxes. On ingestion, that might cause a bit of vomiting, and soap in the eyes is an uncomfortable experience, to say the least.

Water is the cure for both situations: a glassful in the case of an ingestion; a fifteen-minute lukewarm rinse in the case of an eye exposure.

Rust Removers

It takes a tough chemical to dissolve rust, and phosphoric acid is usually the candidate called on. While nowhere nearly as strong as hydrofluoric acid, phosphoric acid can do some serious damage, particularly if sprayed into the eyes. If that happens, rinse the eyes for fifteen to thirty minutes and plan to see a doctor for follow-up. Needless to say, ingestions of concentrated phosphoric acid can be serious. Do not induce vomiting. Dilute with a small glass of water and head to the emergency room.

It's a Fact

- Phosphoric acid is used in low concentrations to add a flavorful zing to some foods, including soft drinks. Maybe that's how some colas got a reputation as rust removers.

Car Cleaners

Cleaning fluids for cars—the kind you mix up with water—generally contain some mildly irritating soaps. If these splash into the eyes, rinse them out for ten to fifteen minutes with lukewarm water. For ingestions, give a glass of milk, water, or juice and expect a short session of vomiting.

Car waxes often contain hydrocarbons—a catch-all term for

petroleum products. Hydrocarbons are in the gasoline family, but it's doubtful that these solid forms could infect the lungs if swallowed. Still, don't induce vomiting. Keep an eye on the person's breathing for about six hours. If anything unusual develops, go to the emergency room. But frankly, it's doubtful you'll see a problem with a small ingestion.

Interior car cleaners—dashboard rejuvenators, for example—contain a variety of ingredients, most commonly silicone. Silicones are nontoxic. Check with your local poison center to see if your car cleaner contains something else.

Car deodorizers—like those little pine trees that hang from the rearview mirror—are impregnated with essential oils: highly concentrated natural products that give off a fragrance as they evaporate. Sucking on one of these will probably irritate the lips and mouth, but there's too little of the essential oil to cause any further problem.

Gasoline and Related Products

One simple rule: Gasoline ingestion = No vomiting.

Believe it or not, you're far better off leaving gasoline in the stomach than vomiting it back up. Gasoline weighs less than many liquids, and if it's forced back up the throat it is likely to float above anything else in the stomach. That gives gasoline a chance to drip into the lungs, where it can set up a sometimes deadly case of chemical pneumonia. Those who swallow gasoline don't necessarily need to report immediately to the emergency room, unless they can't stop coughing or if they develop respiratory symptoms—coughing, wheezing, fever—within six hours after the exposure. Remember: *There is bound to be some initial coughing after a gasoline swallow. But it should clear up quickly and not return. If it does return, or if it never resolves in the first place, that's your cue to go to the emergency room.*

Treatment

Adults have a more well-developed separation between the esophagus and the breathing tubes and so are less likely to get chemical pneumonia from gasoline. Still, anyone who swallows gasoline should do the following:

- Avoid drinking or eating any large amount for about two hours following the exposure. This will minimize the risk of vomiting. After two hours have passed, resume normal eating and drinking.
- Use a small dose of an antacid for heartburn from the gasoline.
- Report immediately to the emergency room if coughing, wheezing, fever, or pain on breathing occurs within six hours of the gasoline ingestion.

Gasoline in the eyes is usually no big deal. Rinse the eyes out with warm water for fifteen minutes. Redness and irritation should abate within an hour. See a doctor if they don't.

Gasoline left on the skin for a long time can cause a burn. Wash it off immediately with soap and warm water.

Siphoning

There's no mouthwash strong enough to combat gasoline breath, a common side effect of swallowing gasoline. Gasoline is extremely volatile, meaning that it readily converts from a liquid to a gaseous state. Thus anyone who swallows gasoline will stink of it for many hours afterward, as gasoline fumes rise from the stomach and exit through the mouth.

A gasoline taste on burping is another common complaint from home siphoners. As long as there is no persistent coughing, gasoline burping is harmless.

Huffing

There is, perhaps, no more desperate form of substance abuse than "huffing." It's also one of the most dangerous. Commonly, a gasoline huffer is a teenager, because gasoline is cheap, it's easy to come by, and nobody asks any questions when you buy it. Gasoline produces a dizzying high that's not unlike the feeling that comes from smoking the first cigarette. As with alcohol, gasoline huffers may become tired after this initial period of euphoria.

What's wrong with huffing gasoline? Lots. First, gasoline is not pure. It's a toxic stew of additives and carbonaceous compounds that can irreversibly damage the brain, causing such symptoms as walking with a stumble. Gasoline also contains a small concentration of benzene, exposure to which over the long run may result in cancer.

It's a Fact

• Don't siphon. Nearly every swallow of gasoline reported to poison control centers is a result of siphoning.

• Until the advent of the automobile, gasoline was considered a nuisance by-product in the manufacture of kerosene and was routinely thrown away.

• In 1913, demand for gasoline outstripped supply, and the United States suffered its first gasoline shortage. The petroleum industry responded by developing a new technique for producing gasoline, called "cracking." Cracking involves the application of heat and pressure to petroleum to "crack" apart chemical bonds and yield more gasoline.

• The earliest home use of gasoline was in stoves in the late 1800s. Back then, gasoline was called "stove naphtha."

• The octane of gasoline has nothing to do with its toxicity. Rather, it is a measure of how efficiently the fuel burns.

• The first oil rush was in the state of Pennsylvania, when Colonel Edwin L. Drake struck oil by drilling in Titusville on August 27, 1859. It took another forty-eight years before the first service station opened.

If gasoline huffers share one characteristic, it's this: They stink. And it is the persistent odor of gasoline that is, perhaps, the most obvious sign of trouble. Anyone suspected of habitually huffing gasoline needs medical evaluation.

Motor Oil

Many products found in the garage start from the same petroleum base as gasoline. In the distillation process, motor oil is drawn off at a different point. As a result it is heavier and, if ingested, less dangerous.

Like gasoline, motor oil can get into the lungs if swallowed, so don't induce vomiting. Instead, restrict food and fluid intake for two hours following the exposure and watch for any signs of a respiratory problem for a total of six hours. You're home free if you see no persistent coughing, wheezing, or fever during that time. It *is* possible to see a touch of diarrhea later as the motor oil passes through the intestines.

Motor oil isn't as irritating to the eyes and skin as gasoline. However, it is never acceptable to allow a petroleum product to stay in contact with the skin for an extended period of time, as damage to the cells could result. So in the case of an exposure to the eyes or skin, rinse thoroughly for ten to fifteen minutes with lukewarm water.

Transmission Fluid

Most brands of transmission fluid and power steering fluid also have a petroleum base. Treat exposures to these the same way you would motor oil.

Gasoline Additives

Many gasoline additives are made of minimally toxic silicones. However, some of these octane boosters and lubricants contain petroleum distillates, so observe the same precautions with these that you would with gasoline. With a large number of gasoline additives on the market, check with the poison center to see what yours contains.

Car Batteries

When you think about it, automobile engines should be exploding all over the place, so loaded are they with reactive fluids and fires. And one of the most volatile chemicals found under the hood is the sulfuric acid inside the battery.

Generally, the biggest risk from a car battery is an explosion brought on by the spark from jumper cables. Sulfuric acid causes burns, true burns. That is, sulfuric acid has such an affinity for water that it tends to char the skin rather than dissolve it. It's this affinity for water that makes sulfuric acid so irritating to the moist tissues of the eyes, nose, and lungs.

> **It's a Fact**
>
> • Asthmatics and those with emphysema or other respiratory problems have a harder time handling sulfuric acid fumes than others.
>
> • Sulfuric acid is one of the main ingredients in smog.

If a car battery explodes in a family member's face, call 911. Smaller exposures, such as a bit of acid in the eye, can initially be handled at home with thorough lukewarm-water flushing, for fifteen to thirty minutes, followed by a medical examination.

Air Bags

The burst of an air bag is usually the sign that a life is about to be saved. But sadly, there is danger in safety: Small children have been killed by air bags. There's another problem with these devices as well: They can sometimes cause burns, both thermal and chemical. Air bags engage via an electrical spark (the thermal burn), which reacts with the chemical sodium azide to produce nitrogen gas. That's what inflates the bag. One by-product of this reaction is the corrosive material sodium hydroxide (the chemical burn). Treatment of these burns depends on severity. Following a traffic accident in which an air bag deploys, be wary of any complaints of burning sensations or the appearance of blisters. Minor burns can be treated at home, but any burn that blisters should be treated by a doctor.

5

The Cellar

Cellars often turn into toxic—not to mention inflammable—museums. From old paint colors to gummed-up tubes of caulk to half-eaten trays of rat poison, the history of our houses can sometimes be traced by the contents of the basement. But often, it's what you *can't* see that's the problem.

Gases

Carbon Monoxide

Every winter, carbon monoxide (CO) makes the news when some unlucky soul succumbs to the fumes from an improperly working heater. While space heaters more commonly cause CO poisoning, a furnace or hot water heater can leak the poisonous gas if an exhaust pipe is broken or if the machine isn't burning its fuel properly.

In the body, carbon monoxide attacks hemoglobin, a molecule found in the blood that transports oxygen to the tissues. The CO, in effect, puts a headlock on the hemoglobin, preventing it from carrying oxygen. The tissues—and that includes organs like the heart and brain—starve.

The problem for homeowners is that carbon monoxide is an insidious killer. You can't smell it, taste it, or see it. And by the time it starts having an effect on you, it's sometimes too late to get away from it. Do yourself a favor. Once a year have your furnace and hot water heater checked by a reputable heating, ventilating, and air-conditioning company. And never use a kerosene-burning space heater without providing adequate ventilation. Even if it's cold, open the windows a crack.

What does carbon monoxide poisoning feel like? In the early stages, or in a house where there's just a small leak, it feels like the stomach flu. You'll usually feel tired, have a headache, maybe even some nausea and vomiting. As the concentration of the deadly gas increases, more fatigue sets in, until you are sleepy and uncoordinated much of the time. A deadly build-up of carbon monoxide causes rapid suffocation.

With small leaks, you'll often find that the headaches and sleepiness you and other family members might suffer while in the house will disappear once you leave. Slowly, the symptoms get worse, however, until you even feel ill *outside* the poisoned home. That's because CO tends to build up in the body the longer you're exposed to it.

The only sure way to know whether you've got carbon monoxide poisoning is to have a test done at the hospital called a carboxyhemoglobin level. It's a simple test that involves pulling a sample of arterial blood—a bit painful, but nothing too traumatic. Based on the results of that test, you may be given 100 percent oxygen through a mask on an outpatient basis or even admitted for overnight observation.

The most severely poisoned will probably be treated in a hyperbaric oxygen chamber. This device sends oxygen molecules into the tissues with such atmospheric force that they push the tightly bound CO molecules from the body's hemoglobin. While hyperbaric treatment can be lifesaving, it can't bring dead tissue back to life. CO poisoning sometimes leaves behind permanent damage to nerve cells and the heart.

Radon

Radon, the other cellar gas you can't see or smell, won't kill you instantly. Rather, it's the long-term effects on the lungs that are of most concern. Even if you've never been a smoker, if you live in a

It's a Fact

• Your pets—mammalian, that is—are a good indication of whether carbon monoxide is making you sick. They, too, will be ill.

• Cigarette smokers usually have a permanent level of carbon monoxide in their blood (now you know another reason why it's bad to smoke).

• Don't worry about electric heat and electric water heaters. They don't give off carbon monoxide.

• If you feel sick every time you travel in your car, have the exhaust system checked. Sometimes carbon monoxide can leak into the passenger cabin.

• Don't rely solely on a carbon monoxide detector to keep your house safe. These have varying degrees of accuracy. To be completely safe, have your furnace checked every year for leaks and proper burn.

• Always check the flue before you light up the fireplace. It should be open and clear to the sky. Remember, any burning material can give off carbon monoxide.

• If a fire breaks out in your home and a family member comes down with symptoms of confusion, headache, drowsiness, and uncoordination even days later, have them checked for carbon monoxide poisoning.

• Heat and hot water systems aren't the only sources of carbon monoxide in the house. Paint strippers, usually made of methylene chloride, give off fumes that the body converts into CO. Always maintain vigorous ventilation when using paint strippers.

house with persistently high radon levels some researchers believe you could develop lung cancer. Others disagree.

Mortgage lenders seem to have come down on the side of the precautionists in the radon argument. Thus, in some areas of the country, a radon test is mandatory before a mortgage lender will allow a home transaction to go through. If the test shows high radon levels, mitigation measures—such as elaborate (and expensive) ventilation systems—might be needed.

Radon is a by-product of uranium, a substance naturally found in soil and rocks. As uranium degrades, a constant process that happens with any radioactive material, it forms several types of radon. The one that enters our homes is called radon-222. If the house is well ventilated, the radon will not stick around and thus won't hurt you.

But radon that's allowed to accumulate breaks down after about four days into radioactive particles that attach themselves to dust. The dust gets inhaled, the lungs get radiated, and cancer has a chance to begin.

How can you tell whether or not you've got radon? Without testing for it, you can't. You can make some educated guesses, though. If your neighbor has a high radon level, chances are you might, too. But that isn't always the case. You need to have your home tested to know for sure whether you've got a radon problem.

Metal Fume Fever

Home welders who fail to use a respirator can develop a syndrome that feels like food poisoning and the flu wrapped up in one miserable package. It's called metal fume fever and is the result of inhaling the freshly produced oxides of copper, zinc, and other metals. It's not a serious disorder, it only feels like one. If you develop metal fume fever, take antacids for nausea and nonprescription analgesics (acetaminophen, aspirin, ibuprofen) for the aches and pains. It usually resolves after one or two days.

Poisons and Baits

Rat Poison

You say you're in a panic because your child has eaten a few pellets of rat poison? Relax. There's no need to panic. Here's why:

Today's rat poisons are usually made of brodifacoum, a chemical that prevents the rodent's blood from coagulating. So the rat bleeds to death. Brodifacoum takes several days to have an effect on human blood, and the amount of brodifacoum in rat poisons is small—usually about .005 percent. Therefore, it takes a substantial ingestion of pellets to cause poisoning in a child.

How substantial? It depends how much the person weighs. But suffice to say, most ingestions of brodifacoum rat poison do *not* result in symptoms, because not enough of the compound is ingested. Why is this so? Brodifacoum pellets look like they might taste good—usually they're a bright green or blue color—but they don't. So most children lose interest in them quickly.

Always call the poison center after a rat poison ingestion and be prepared to answer this question: How many pellets did your child eat? Don't make a wild guess, try for an educated one that you can sleep with comfortably. If you really don't know, say so.

Not every poison center agrees on what is and isn't a toxic level of pellets, but you can be reasonably sure it's a lot higher than you think. Low levels—a few pellets—are left untreated, medium levels—say ten to twenty pellets—might be treated at home with ipecac syrup, and unknown or high levels go to the emergency room for a stomach

It's a Fact

- Poison centers will sometimes advise watching for signs of unusual bleeding after a rat poison ingestion—from the nose, the gums, and under the skin as bruises. With low- to medium-level ingestions these symptoms are very unlikely.
- While brodifacoum is not the only rat poison available, others, including warfarin and the indanediones, work the same way—by causing the animal to bleed to death.
- Rat poisons probably got their fearsome reputation because of the compounds formerly used: strychnine and an extremely toxic chemical called sodium fluoroacetate. These are no longer sold for home use, but if you own an old house, clean out your cellar! There may be a stray box lying about.

washout followed by a dose of activated charcoal and a follow-up appointment for a blood check.

Ant and Roach Traps

Look at the containers these come in, such as Combat and Amdro, and you can see why they cause few problems on ingestion. First, the containers are small. Second, they're hard to break open. Third, there's only a small amount of poison in each trap. And finally, some of these poisons are minimally toxic—hydramethylnon, for example. It's almost impossible for a child to get poisoned by an ant trap.

It's a Fact

- Keep dogs and cats away from ant bait disks, because they may contain dog food to lure the ants in. It's not so much that the poison inside is a problem for the animal; it's that they might choke on the disk.

Paint

Maybe your cellar looks like mine: great numbers of paint cans stacked on shelves and on the floor, the only thing each having in common being a half-moon shape paint drip dried to the side of the can. In general, the older the paint, the greater the possibility it may contain lead. Discard old paint cans—they're nothing but trouble—making sure you follow safe disposal laws where you live.

Latex Paints

These days, most homeowners use latex paint products inside the house. They're easy to clean up with water, have little odor, and—even though they're made up of a stew of poisonous materials—have low toxicity when ingested. There's just not enough of any one poison in a can of latex paint to be of concern. So if a brush licking occurs, or a child dips a finger into latex paint to see if it tastes as good as it looks, don't worry about it.

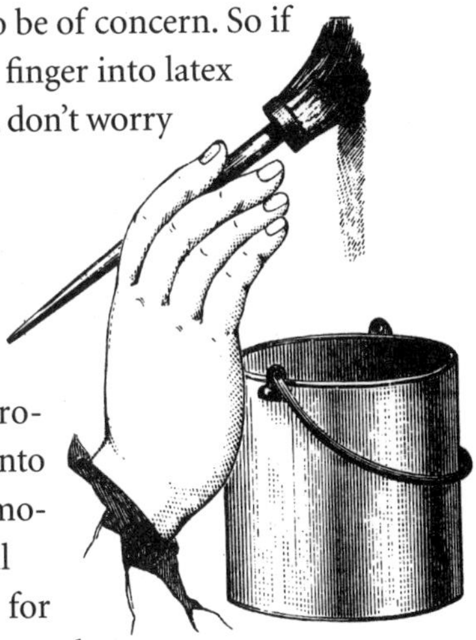

Oil-based Paints

These are a bit more problematic, owing to their petroleum base. As with gasoline, it's possible some of the petroleum solvent in an oil paint could slide into the lungs if swallowed and set up pneumonia. So don't induce vomiting with oil paints. Instead, restrict food and fluid for two hours, and watch for any respiratory problems for six: coughing, wheezing, or fever. If any of these develop, head to the emergency room. If nothing occurs after this six-hour observation period, you're home free.

Lead Paints

Lead paint hasn't been available for twenty years, so it's unlikely even a home paint museum will have a can of it lying around. The main lead danger in homes these days is from the ingestion of lead paint chips or lead paint dust. If lead paint is intact—that is, if it's firmly affixed to the wall with no peeling occurring—it's not an immediate hazard.

Eating a chip or two of lead paint is not likely to cause a significant problem. But continous ingestion allows lead to accumulate in the body, especially in the teeth and bones. The effect on the brain and nervous system is most troublesome. Children exposed to chronic low levels of lead develop difficulty in concentrating. They are often tired and show a lack of initiative. Sometimes lead may affect the nerves of the legs and arms, so that the limbs function in a sluggish manner. With serious lead poisoning, "lead colic" develops: intense, gripping bouts of pain in the abdomen caused by intestinal spasms. (In low-level lead exposures, the only gastrointestinal symptom may be bouts of constipation.)

The more dramatic—and more rapidly fatal—type of lead

It's a Fact

- Lead has been blamed for the fall of the Roman Empire, but it's never been proven as an absolute cause. The Romans did use lead in a number of ways—to line pipes and flasks and as an additive to wine to retard spoilage.
- There is no such thing as a lead-free environment. Given the preponderance of ores in the earth that contain lead, we probably all get some lead in our water.
- Paint is not the only home source of lead. Glazed earthenware containers that have not been subject to high-heat curing can leach lead when in contact with acidic foods. Play it safe: Never eat from an earthenware container produced by an amateur potter. Those produced commercially in the United States are usually fine.
- Lead poisoning is also known as "plumbism"; the chemical symbol for lead is Pb.
- Fewer newspaper inks contain lead these days, so chewing on a piece of *The Daily Rag* isn't especially hazardous, as long as it's not habitual. The same is true for magazines.
- Lead objects swallowed whole, such as fishing sinkers, are not an immediate hazard except for choking. If they make it to the stomach, they can be allowed to pass through the system. However, they must pass out of the body or they may begin leaching lead.
- One reason you might feel tired from lead poisoning is that lead causes anemia. Ferrous sulfate, a form of iron, is often prescribed to correct that problem.

poisoning is an acute large exposure, such as might occur in industry. But even long-term, low-level lead exposure can explode into a serious illness if, for example, lead is liberated into the system from multiple broken bones.

Most childhood lead poisonings are of the insidious variety. They creep up with few obvious signs or symptoms and only get detected by a blood test. If you live in an old house where there might be lead paint on the walls, and there's a risk your child may have eaten some chips, have a lead test done. Some poison centers even recommend using ipecac for a few paint chips. Needless to say, swallowing liquid lead paint is extremely hazardous and might warrant emergency-room treatment.

Long-term treatment for lead poisoning depends on the blood test results, and each year, it seems, the government lowers the level considered to be toxic. At very low lead levels, observation and retesting are common solutions, along with ending all possibility of further exposure—removing lead paint, for example. The most serious cases of lead poisoning require using drugs that bind the metal up. These are powerful drugs that cause numerous side effects, so you want to avoid having to use one. Penicillamine is one example of such a drug; others include EDTA and BAL.

Paint Clean-up Products

Here's another good reason to use latex paints whenever possible: They clean up with soap and water. For oil-based paints you need to use a toxic and usually inflammable chemical like mineral spirits or turpentine.

Mineral Spirits

Like gasoline, mineral spirits, when swallowed, can drip into the lungs and set up chemical pneumonia. By now, you know the drill. For a swallow of mineral spirits *do not induce vomiting.* Instead, watch for persistent coughing, wheezing, fever, or any other sign that might indicate inflammation in the lungs. For the first two hours of observation, give little or nothing by mouth to avoid stimulating vomiting. If six hours go by without symptoms, you can stop worrying.

Turpentine

Turpentine ingestions are a double-edged sword. Turpentine is extremely toxic if left in the stomach, but extremely toxic to the lungs if vomited up. So, how to handle it? First, if it's a very small ingestion—a taste, for example—it's probably best just to observe at home for signs of pneumonia. If any respiratory symptoms occur within six hours, head to the emergency room. If it's a larger ingestion—say, anything greater than a teaspoonful in a young child—it's probably best to go to the emergency room without delay. Turpentine exerts its toxic effects on the stomach and intestines (it's very irritating), on the heart, and on the brain (it causes seizures).

It's a Fact

- One home remedy calls for the use of turpentine on poison ivy. Don't do it. Turpentine can actually burn and blister the skin. That's a whole lot worse than a case of poison ivy.
- Turpentine, derived from pine trees, is an aromatic substance with a pleasing odor. But excessive inhalation of turpentine fumes can cause dizziness and irritation to the mucus membranes.

Only vigorous flushing will stop the burning pain of turpentine in the eyes or on the skin. For the eyes, flush for up to thirty minutes with lukewarm water. The eyes will be red after this flushing but should return to normal within another thirty minutes. If they remain extremely red, or there's pain or trouble seeing, head to the emergency room.

Other Brush and Paint Products

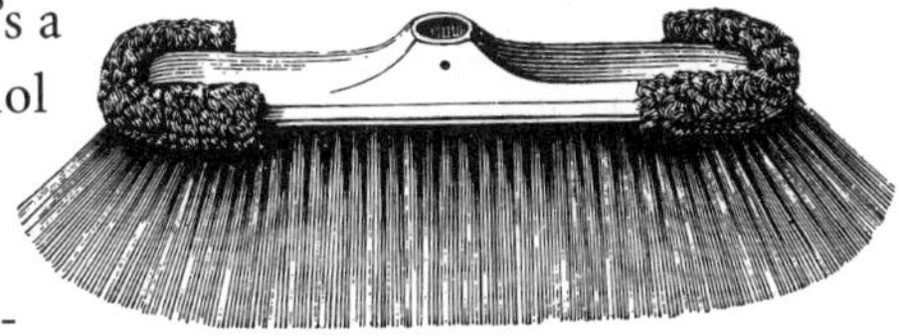

Beware denatured alcohol. It's a mixture of highly toxic methanol and ethanol, and any amount could be poisonous.

Small amounts of pure acetone—a taste, for example—rarely cause a problem. But severe drowsiness can occur with larger amounts. Try to estimate the number of teaspoonfuls of acetone ingested, and know your child's weight when you call the poison center.

Products labeled "paint thinners" are often nothing more than mineral spirits, but "lacquer thinners" can contain toxic additives like methanol and toluene.

Japan drier, used to speed up the drying time for oil-based paints, contains hydrocarbons. Ingestions of Japan drier should be treated the same as with mineral spirits.

MEK, sometimes used to thin paint or clean brushes, is methyl ethyl ketone. Left on the skin, MEK can be absorbed and might cause dizziness, drowsiness, or worse. Like mineral spirits, MEK, if swallowed, can get into the lungs and cause pneumonia. Don't induce vomiting. Call the poison center.

When you use xylene as a paint thinner, crack open the windows—it's mainly poisonous when inhaled. Xylene fumes cause headaches and dizziness. It's also extremely irritating to the skin and eyes.

Grease and oil dissolvers sometimes find their way to the paint shelf. One popular chemical used as a grease remover is trichloroethane, or TCE. TCE damages the skin, so wash it off quickly. Also, keep a window open when using TCE as its fumes cause dizziness and even heart problems at a high concentration.

Wallpaper strippers fall into two categories: extremely dangerous and harmless. The newer "safe" strippers contain an enzyme product to dissolve paint and wallpaper. They may be irritating to the eyes and skin but are generally safe. Older and stronger strippers contain methanol. Any ingestion of methanol is an emergency.

Don't worry too much about linseed oil. It might cause diarrhea, but little else.

Old cans of shellac, polyurethane, and wood stains commonly clutter the shelves in many cellars. For the most part, these are petroleum-based products, meaning they have the same potential toxicity as mineral spirits—chemical pneumonia if they get into the lungs. But with so many of these products on the market, check with a poison center to be sure yours fits into the hydrocarbon category.

It's a Fact

- Water-based stains, often sold as "safe" alternatives to petroleum-based products, sometimes contain poisonous compounds similar to ethylene glycol.
- Wood conditioners, used to make stain spread more evenly, may contain propylene glycol. Small ingestions of propylene glycol are harmless.

Wall and Concrete Cleaners

Muriatic Acid

It takes a tough chemical to work on concrete, and muriatic acid is no pussycat. Actually, muriatic acid is simply another name for hydrochloric acid, the same caustic fluid secreted by our stomachs to break down food.

The muriatic acid you buy at the hardware store is a bit more concentrated than what's in your gut. If swallowed, it could burn a hole through the stomach. *Don't induce vomiting.* Sip a glass of water slowly. Gravity carries acids to the stomach, where they pool and cause damage. Water weakens the acid by diluting it. But dilution may not be enough of a treatment, so be prepared to go to the hospital.

Muriatic acid in the eyes is an extreme emergency. Flush with lukewarm water for thirty minutes, then head to the hospital. For the skin, do a similarly long irrigation. Head for the hospital if blisters appear or the skin begins to peel.

Trisodium Phosphate

Trisodium phosphate, or TSP, used to clean walls before painting, is, like muriatic acid, corrosive. However, because it's an alkaline corrosive (versus an acidic one), you're more likely to see burns develop in the mouth and throat than in the stomach. Still, some of the same rules apply. No vomiting. Dilute with sips from a small glass of water. But before scooting off to the emergency room, look for symptoms. If blisters have popped up inside the mouth, or if there's trouble swallowing, or speaking, or excessive drooling, by all means go to the hospital. Keep in mind that burns from alkaline corrosives can take several hours to develop. For eye exposures, rinse thoroughly with lukewarm water for fifteen to thirty minutes, then see a doctor.

Laundry Room

In many homes, one part of the cellar serves as the laundry room, and it's a common site for childhood poisonings. Fortunately, most of the products we use to wash clothes have low toxicity.

Bleach

"My baby swallowed bleach!" It's perhaps the most common complaint poison control centers hear. It's a mystery why children have such an affection for bleach. It smells terrible, tastes worse, and isn't even a pretty color. The probable reason is availability. Parents tend to dispense bleach from those heavy white containers into drink-size cups. To a child, bleach looks like water. After a good swallow of bleach, children will probably cough, choke, scream, and even vomit. But bleach ingestions look worse than they actually are. Give a few ounces of water, milk, or juice. Within a few minutes, the fluid will stimulate vomiting. That's normal. As soon as the stomach has cleared itself of the bleach, the vomiting will stop. *Do not give ipecac syrup after a bleach ingestion.* Vomiting will occur naturally—and if it doesn't, there's no pressing need to get the bleach out of the stomach. It's not that poisonous.

On the other hand, there *is* a pressing need to rinse out bleach that has splashed into the eyes; it's extremely irritating and could even cause damage. Do a fifteen-minute flush with lukewarm water. In some cases, a follow-up examination by a doctor might be necessary.

Bleach, Ammonia, and Vinegar

Nothing can wreck a good bathroom-cleaning session more than combining bleach and ammonia. They don't even have to be mixed in the same container to cause a reaction; the mere presence of an opened bottle of each might result in a chemical reaction that creates highly poisonous chloramine gas. This gas combines with the water naturally present in the tissues of the eyes, nose, throat, and lungs and forms hydrochloric acid. And that, folks, can inflame the lungs. The result: chemical pneumonia.

Never mix bleach with acidic materials, either. Some homemakers use vinegar or lemon juice as cleaners. That's fine. But mixing them with bleach might cause the release of poisonous chlorine gas, which can have the same effect on the lungs.

Even using bleach alone carries risks. Symptoms of bleach inhalation include a productive cough (one that produces mucus) and a feeling of heaviness in the chest. These symptoms could indicate inflammation in the lungs and, if severe, might require medical treatment.

It's a Fact

• Never clean a child's potty using bleach, unless you have first rinsed it out with water. Urine contains ammonia, and the two will react to form chloramine gas.

• Bleach is one of the most important relief ingredients following a natural disaster. After a hurricane, sewage systems often overflow, causing contamination of drinking water supplies. Adding a bit of bleach to contaminated water insures that harmful bacteria are killed. A small amount—ten drops added to one gallon of water—will kill off any disease-causing microbes.

• Never bleach the hair using laundry bleach. It will burn the scalp and may drip into the eyes. (See Dyes in chapter 6.)

• The trade name Clorox is a combination of chlorine and oxygen, two of the necessary ingredients to make bleach. It's also a shorthand description of how bleach works: oxidation via chlorine.

• The most powerful bleaching agent in the world rises above us every day: the sun. The ancient Hebrews and Egyptians bleached fabrics by leaving them in the sun.

Laundry Detergents

Most laundry detergents, liquid or powder, are relatively safe. But a few contain ingredients that could be corrosive: sodium carbonate and sodium silicate.

Even these, however, rarely cause burns when swallowed, so the treatment for every laundry detergent is the same: Give a glass of milk, water, or juice and expect a short session of vomiting as the stomach clears itself of the soap. Some laundry detergents might induce a bit of diarrhea; others, allergic symptoms like a scratchy throat. But the important symptoms to watch for are difficulty in swallowing and heavy drooling. See a doctor if these occur; they might indicate a throat burn.

It's a Fact

- Specialty fabric cleaners—liquids for wool, for example—usually contain nothing more than soaps.
- Fabric softeners are made of strong detergents. While a throat burn is unlikely with a swallow of fabric softener, be alert for difficulty in swallowing and heavy drooling. See a doctor if these occur.
- Keep the windows open when you're using home spot removers, as some contain the toxic solvent trichloroethane, which, when inhaled, causes dizziness. Others—Spray 'n Wash, for example—are less toxic.
- The main ingredients in home clothing dyes are salt and baking soda. A taste of dye is no big deal. Larger amounts may require treatment, depending on the victim's age and weight. Also, some clothing dyes cause diarrhea.
- Spray starches are nontoxic if eaten, but an intentional inhalation from the can could trigger a heart attack from the propellants.
- Don't worry about dryer sheets. They're impregnated with fabric softeners that might irritate the mouth, if chewed, but do little else.

6

The Bathroom

Keeping all that porcelain and tile sparkling clean requires the use of some pretty nasty chemicals. And that's really where we run into the most trouble in the bathroom—with cleaners that scour mildew and mold from grouting, chemicals that bust through clogged drain lines, and acids that eat away stubborn toilet stains. But first, let's take a look at personal hygiene products, which, when compared to the others, are no sweat.

Washing Up

Shampoo

It's distressing when a child starts vomiting after a swallow of shampoo—many times it will come up as suds. Not to worry, though. Shampoos are mild soap formulations that only irritate the stomach. Give a glass of fluid after a shampoo ingestion and expect mild vomiting to occur shortly thereafter.

Let a bit of that "no more tears" shampoo slide into the eyes, and you'll realize there's no such thing as a tearless shampoo. But shampoos won't harm the eyes, only irritate them. If you're in the bathtub when it happens, turn on a slow, lukewarm shower stream and encourage the child to look up at it. The eyes need about ten minutes of rinsing to get the shampoo out. They'll stay red for a good half hour afterward, but there should be continuous improvement. If not, see a doctor.

Soap

Remember the disciplinary ritual of getting your mouth washed out with soap? Well, it's best to find another way to discourage cursing, as soap irritates the inside of the mouth and causes gagging and vomiting. Your first priority is to be sure the child isn't choking on a chunk of soap. Otherwise, the treatment for an accidental soap ingestion is the same as for shampoo: dilute and observe.

Cream Rinses and Conditioners

Cream rinses and conditioners came into vogue during the 1970s, and they've never left us. These products consist of fats, waxes, and oils, which are not toxic, and "cationic" detergents, which are. Normally, cationic detergents are more irritating than the "anionic" detergents you find in soaps and shampoos, but when it comes to hair conditioners, the worst you're likely to see

It's a Fact

• These days, everything from fruit extracts to wheat germ to vitamins has made its way into shampoos. Before World War II shampoos were a bit simpler; they consisted of soap and water.

• We may take soap for granted, but it's an amazing substance that acts as a bridge between grease and water—dissolving the former so it can be lifted off by the latter.

• Some brands of deodorant soap once contained hexachlorophene, a chemical banned from over-the-counter use in the early 1970s for fear it harmed the central nervous system.

• Medicated shampoos for dandruff, psoriasis, and itchy scalp contain toxic ingredients like benzocaine and coal tar, but small amounts are not likely to cause a problem. Treat the same as you would any other shampoo ingestion.

is vomiting and a bit of diarrhea. Treat ingestions of these as you would shampoo: dilute and observe.

Bath Gels

Kids love to bite into bath gels, those round orbs of colored liquid that dissolve in warm water. Fortunately, they're not harmful. Bath gels might contain a small amount of mineral oil, plus some soaps and a fragrance. There's a possibility of light vomiting, but little else. Give a glass of fluid and observe. The same generally goes for bath salts and bath cubes.

In general—and there are numerous brands, so check with your poison center—liquid bath preparations, such as bubble bath or body gels, are minimally toxic. Some contain oils and fats, so loose stools may develop or perhaps a touch of vomiting.

Hair Care

Home Permanents and Relaxers

The nastiest hair products on the market are those used to create perms, especially hair straighteners and relaxers. These usually contain some type of corrosive ingredient, such as sodium hydroxide, and it's not unusual for burns to occur in both children and adults. In kids, it's usually from taking a taste; in adults, it's because the perm has dripped into the eyes or been left on the scalp too long.

Cognizant of these possibilities, the manufacturers of home permanents and relaxers have kept the corrosive concentrations relatively low, giving these products a pH around 12: highly irritating but not necessarily corrosive. Still, children frequently sustain blisters and burns to the lips and inside the mouth with home perm solutions, and burns could develop in the throat if enough is swallowed.

After an ingestion, check the mouth and lips carefully. If you see blisters, peeling skin, or anything else that looks like a burn, go to the emergency room. Otherwise, wash out the mouth, give a small glass of water or milk, and observe for difficulty swallowing, excessive drooling, or a change in the way the voice sounds. Remember, these symptoms could take several hours to develop. Seek medical help if they do.

Treat a corrosive perm drip to the eyes with a thorough thirty-minute lukewarm water rinse. Plan on seeing a doctor following the rinse.

Severe burns to the scalp and skin are possible from use of a home permanent. See a doctor if these burns occur.

Another type of perm—sometimes found in cold wave relaxers—is thioglycolate. It's not quite as dangerous as sodium hydroxide, but it's still capable of causing burns, especially when left too long on the scalp. Follow the same treatment guidelines as for the other perms, but expect less of a problem.

It's a Fact

- Depilatories—products to remove unwanted hair from the body—are formulated in much the same way as perms and relaxers, with thioglycolate and corrosive alkaline chemicals.

Dyes

The same chemical has been used in modern hair dying for almost a hundred years: paraphenylenediamine. It's extremely toxic. Aside from occasionally causing severe allergic reactions, paraphenylenediamine can damage the kidneys if ingested, even in relatively small amounts. Hydrogen peroxide hair dyes are generally safer; they're also found in products to dye unwanted body hair.

For paraphenylenediamine hair dye ingestions, call the poison center and plan to go to the emergency room. Hydrogen peroxide dye ingestions can usually be treated at home with a glass of fluid, but consult a poison center first.

Fresh Breath and Healthy Teeth

Toothpaste

One of the most toxic ingredients you'll find in the bathroom is fluoride. Excessive fluoride not only corrodes the lining of the stomach, it also affects the function of the heart and other organs. It's possible that ingesting toothpaste might cause fluoride poisoning, but before you start locking up the Crest, be assured that it would take a *lot* of toothpaste to cause a problem. Here's why.

Most fluoride toothpastes contain just 1.1 milligrams of fluoride per gram or about 5 milligrams in a teaspoonful. That's not a very high concentration of fluoride. So it would take a rather large ingestion of toothpaste to result in fluoride poisoning. Also, there's a soapy element to toothpaste that could very well stimulate vomiting before significant absorption of fluoride occurs.

So, for all intents and purposes, toothpaste does not present a serious hazard, as far as fluoride goes. It's much the same story with over-the-counter fluoride rinses. While it's possible to ingest enough of a rinse to cause toxicity, it's unlikely any child would do so.

Mouthwash

Nonfluoride mouthwashes are another story. Desperate alcoholics sometimes buy bottles of highly antiseptic and bitter mouthwashes because they contain about 20 percent alcohol. Better-tasting mouthwashes—

It's a Fact

• The first fluoride toothpaste on the market was Crest with Fluoristan, introduced in 1956.

• Ready to gag? Even into the eighteenth century, urine was used as a mouthwash in Europe.

• Dairy products are your first line of defense against fluoride, as calcium prevents fluoride from being absorbed. Barring a huge ingestion, giving a glass of milk or some ice cream relieves the upset stomach that can result from excessive fluoride.

that is, those more appealing to children—have less alcohol but still contain a higher concentration than that found in many wines.

In general, there's no big worry about a swallow of mouthwash, but with several ounces—an amount you might find in a paper bathroom cup—you might run into trouble if a child is doing the drinking. With an ingestion that large, give a sweet drink, such as fruit juice or punch. Sugar helps offset a drop in blood sugar that normally occurs when children drink alcoholic beverages. Observe for sixty minutes. During that time, you're looking for signs of drunkenness: an unsteady gait, fatigue, giddiness. If you see any of these symptoms, go to the emergency room. Some parents find it amusing to see such tipsiness. *It's not funny.* Drunkenness is dangerous in a child. Alcohol drives down blood sugar levels, and that means some cells—particularly brain cells—can starve.

Denture Cleaners

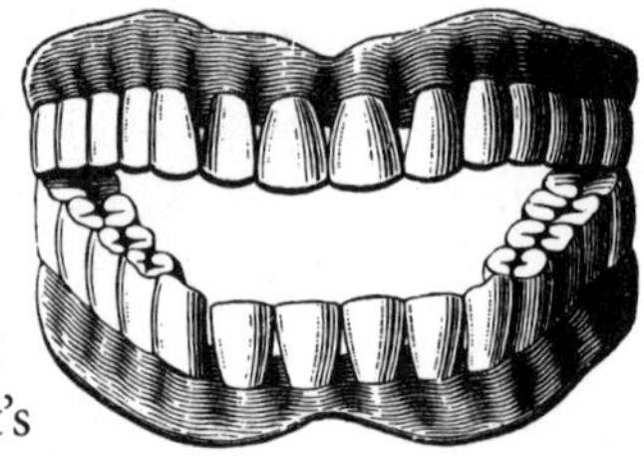

Large fizzy denture-cleaning tablets, if swallowed whole, will almost certainly produce a stomachache—in fact, it's possible that the gas these tablets release could perforate the stomach. Tempering that possibility, however, is the fact that it's difficult to swallow one of these tablets. The second that moisture comes in contact with one, it starts to fizz and froth. And because these contain some soapy materials, vomiting is possible. Call the poison center if an ingestion actually occurs. But that would be unusual.

More Personal Hygiene

Taking a bite out of an underarm deodorant bar (or tasting a bit of a deodorant spray or liquid) might cause some vomiting, but it's nothing serious. Give a glass of milk, water, or juice. These products irritate the stomach.

Contact Lens Products

Common sense will tell you that anything meant to come in contact with the eye can't be very toxic, and that's certainly true of most contact lens solutions and cleaners. One exception is effervescent enzyme tablets, which can irritate the stomach. Give a glass of fluid if one of these tablets is swallowed and observe for possible vomiting.

> **It's a Fact**
>
> • Even if you prefer to use a spray underarm deodorant, keep an unscented solid in the house that contains aluminum. An underarm solid rubbed on a poison ivy rash or an insect sting relieves itching.
>
> • There is little difference in toxicity between underam deodorants and antiperspirants. Treat each with a small glass of fluid and expect minor vomiting.

Yes, there are people out there—crazy people, I might add—who wet their contact lenses by placing them on their tongue. Sometimes the lenses are swallowed. A hard lenses could get caught in the throat and cause choking. But the soft and semisoft varieties will probably dissolve in the stomach. They're harmless.

Fever Thermometers

When broken open, fever thermometers release unruly globules of mercury. Trying to pick these up can be like playing with a toxicological Rubik's cube: Every time you get one of the globules in your hand, it splits into three more pieces that roll away.

Mercury *is* toxic. But thermometer mercury can't be absorbed if swallowed. It passes right through the system and is excreted unchanged in the feces, so poison centers consider thermometer mercury nonpoisonous.

There is one warning: If someone has a perforation in the intestinal tract, thermometer mercury could be transformed into a form that's more poisonous by coming in contact with certain bodily fluids. Still, the amount of mercury in a thermometer is exceedingly small (0.3 milliliter), and it's highly unlikely to cause a problem. Actually, swallowing the glass from a broken thermometer is more dangerous than swallowing the mercury. Small pieces of glass will pass through the intestinal tract without causing damage, provided a normal diet is maintained. But see a doctor if a sizable piece of glass has been swallowed, and never induce vomiting after a glass ingestion.

It's a Fact

- Mercury globules can break down into small particles or vapor when heated, left out in the air, or vacuumed. These can be inhaled, and that might be dangerous. To pick up mercury, soak a paper towel with water and blot it up. Or immobilize the droplets with hair spray and pick them up with a paper towel.

Beard Care Products

The most dangerous beard care product is the razor. If you can keep that away from the kids you've got most of the shaving line licked. A taste of shaving cream is like a taste of shampoo; it might stimulate mild vomiting. Just give a small glass of fluid. Styptic pencils contain a mild astringent that's low in toxicity. If a piece is swallowed, mild vomiting might occur.

Splash on an aftershave lotion and you'll enjoy a cooling effect on the skin, thanks to the alcohol it contains. As with mouthwash, an ingestion of aftershave lotion can be deadly to a child because of the alcohol. Fortunately, aftershave lotions taste awful, and it's difficult to imagine anyone guzzling down a significant amount (though it happens with alcoholics).

If you suspect that might've happened in a child, give a sweet drink and observe for drowsiness, giddiness, and other signs of drunkeness for sixty minutes. If nothing happens within that time, nothing's likely to happen. If you do see signs of inebriation, go immediately to the emergency room.

Aftershave splashed into the eyes feels like fire. Despite the pain, alcohol won't harm the eyes—it only irritates them. Immediately begin rinsing with lukewarm water and continue doing so for about fifteen minutes. Crying is excellent therapy, as well, so never counsel a child to stop crying after such an accident. After you finish rinsing, the eyes will be red, but over the course of about forty-five minutes they should at least begin to clear up. If they don't, see a doctor.

Cleaning Up the Bathroom

Tile Cleaners

There are two types of detergents commonly used in the home. Anionic detergents are the mild kind you find in soaps and shampoos. These work well for light-duty cleaning. But when it comes to things like removing soap scum, you need something stronger. That's where the cationic detergents come in to play.

Just as cationic detergents have the power to dissolve soap scum, so too can they do a job on human tissue. In fact, some of the more popular soap scum removers have pH values nearly as strong as oven cleaner.

Treatment for a skin burn from a cationic detergent is simple: Irrigate the area with lukewarm water for a good fifteen minutes. If blistering or skin damage appears—or if pain doesn't dissipate—see a doctor. In the eyes, rinse for thirty minutes with lukewarm water, then see a doctor no matter how you're feeling.

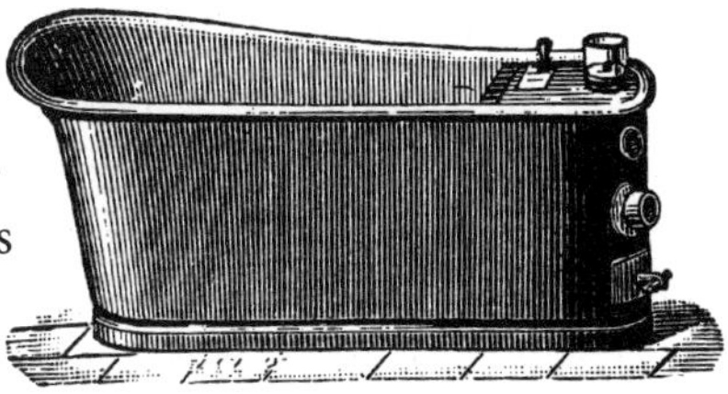

Needless to say, ingesting a tile cleaner can be disastrous. But before you trot off to the emergency room, examine the mouth. If there are blisters, redness, or peeling skin, by all means head to the hospital. But if everything looks clear, just observe for a few hours at home. If there's any difficulty swallowing or speaking, or if excessive drooling occurs, go to the hospital.

Straight mildew removers usually contain bleach, which is less toxic than cationic detergents. For ingestions of a bleach mildew remover, give a glass of fluid and watch for possible vomiting.

Toilet Bowl Cleaners

Here's another opportunity for a chemical burn. Toilet bowl cleaners often contain acids. In fact, crystalline bowl cleaners sometimes have a pH as low as 1. That's highly acidic and highly dangerous. Follow the same treatment recommendations as for tile cleaners, except give a small glass of water to dilute the acid down. Always check the product with the poison center, however, as some bowl cleaners might contain simple (and comparatively harmless) detergents instead.

Toilet Bowl Deodorizers

There's a good reason why those toilet bowl cakes that hang over the side of the bowl smell like mothballs. They're made of the same material: paradichlorobenzene (PDB). A small ingestion of PDB—say, anything up to a couple of mothball-sized chunks—should cause no problems. More than that, and you may need to use ipecac syrup or even go to the emergency room. But in general, PDB has low toxicity. (A tip: When you call the poison center about a toilet bowl deodorizer ingestion, try to phrase the amount eaten in terms of mothball-sized pieces.)

Liquid toilet deodorizers are the bottles you mount in the toilet tank behind the bowl. Most are made up of simple soaps and dyes and are minimally toxic when ingested. Plus, they're usually ingested dilute: Children have a fascination with toilet function, and bluish water only heightens that interest. For an ingestion of "blue" toilet water, simply dilute further with a glass of water, milk, or juice. Vomiting might occur, but it's not likely.

It's a Fact

• Toilet bowl water might be toxic if it contains bacteria from fecal matter. Any child who develops diarrhea, fever, cramps, or other symptoms of food poisoning following a toilet water ingestion should be treated by a doctor.

Drain Openers

We lose, what, about a hundred hairs a day? Well, some of us a bit more than that, maybe. In any case, these hairs have nowhere to go when you're taking a shower other than down the drain. Throw in some soapsuds and shampoo, and you've got a gluey, impenetrable mass. Enter the drain openers: powerful corrosive products that burn their way through clots of hair.

Drain openers are the most dangerous product you'll find in the bathroom; when swallowed, some forms of drain opener—thick liquids, for example—are almost guaranteed to cause a burn in the throat. It's a medical emergency when a drain cleaner is swallowed or gets into the eyes, but there are a few things you can do at home before going to the hospital. For the eyes, do a vigorous rinse for thirty minutes with lukewarm water. For an ingestion, wash out the mouth with a wet cloth. Have the victim, if old enough, swish water and spit several times. Do not give anything to drink or eat, as this may stimulate vomiting. *No matter how well a person feels following a drain opener ingestion or eye exposure, see a doctor.*

Unless you see blistering or extreme irritation, treat skin exposures at home by thoroughly rinsing the area with lukewarm water. However, if the drain opener was splashed to a sensitive area—the genitals or face, for example—see a doctor.

Because drain openers are usually poured through standing water, little attention is paid to the toxic, irritating fumes these products give off. But they can be a problem, so maintain adequate ventilation when using a drain cleaner. And before you resort to Liquid Plumr or Drano, why not consider a nontoxic method for clearing the trap? Use a plunger.

It's a Fact

- The most destructive drain openers are the concentrated liquids. Dilute drain openers or solid crystals are still dangerous, but less so.

Tub and Toilet Caulk

Most caulking materials are largely made of the same thing as chalk: calcium carbonate. As such, they're nontoxic if ingested. You might also find caulks containing all sorts of poisonous solvents, including glycols and hydrocarbons. Usually, these are present in such a small quantity that they're not a problem.

One general rule to follow after a caulk ingestion: don't induce vomiting. Check with a poison center on whether your caulk contains toxic ingredients. Even if it does, in most cases you'll be advised to simply observe for excessive drowsiness or respiratory symptoms: coughing, wheezing, shortness of breath. But frankly, caulks contain such small amounts of poison that it would be unusual to see *any* symptoms develop.

7

The Bedroom and Home Office

There's a blurry line dividing what's usually found in the bedroom and bathroom, so if you didn't find what you're looking for in the previous chapter, chances are you'll find it here. And since many families these days run home businesses from a bedroom, there are a few home office products you should know about as well.

Dolling Up

Whether its rouge, eye shadow, lipstick, or foundation, cosmetics share one common trait: They're nontoxic. Mostly made up of fats, oils, and waxes, these products, if ingested in quantity, might cause some diarrhea. But there's hardly much opportunity for that to happen, as cosmetics are normally packaged in the smallest of containers. So if it's a cosmetic that goes on the skin, you've usually got nothing to worry about.

Painted Nails

Nail polish is like paint: It contains lots of things that could be dangerous, but there's so little of each ingredient, and they're packaged in such small, inaccessible bottles, that they're considered nontoxic.

Nail polish removers are another story, especially the ones that contain acetone. Acetone ingestions, if large enough, can cause drowsiness all the way to a coma. But most ingestions won't result in such dire symptoms. In fact, you will probably see no symptoms at all if the ingestion is small—say, a taste or a swallow. Give a glass of fluid and observe for a few hours. If sudden unexplainable drowsiness occurs during that time, go immediately to the emergency room.

If you've got children in the house, you're better off forsaking the faster action of an acetone nail polish remover for the relative safety of one that contains ethyl acetate, a simple irritant. Ingestions of ethyl acetate might result in a sore throat and mouth, and possibly some vomiting, but it's less toxic than acetone. Dilute with a glass of water, milk, or juice.

Any type of nail polish remover will irritate the eyes, so treat an accidental splash with a fifteen-minute lukewarm-water irrigation. Redness in the eyes should clear within an hour of the rinsing. If it doesn't, see a doctor.

Smelling Good

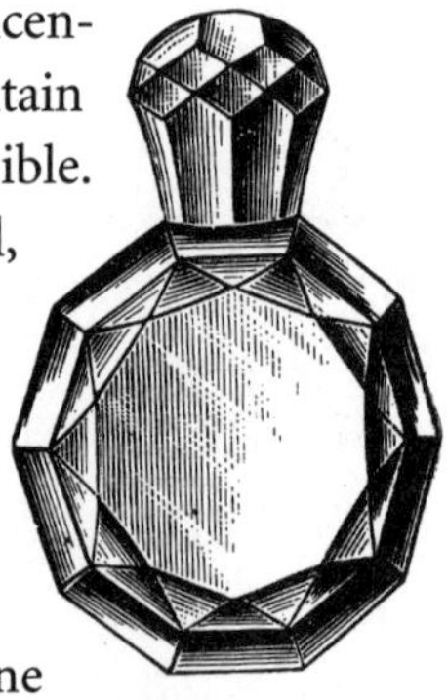

Perfumes and colognes contain high concentrations of alcohol. Fortunately, they also contain numerous agents that make them taste terrible. So most perfume ingestions tend to be small, resulting in no symptoms whatsoever.

Don't panic over a swallow of perfume by a child. Instead, give a glass of fruit juice or another sugar-filled drink (a couple of teasponfuls of sugar mixed with water if you've got nothing else), and observe for one hour. You're looking for signs of drunkenness—typically, drowsiness and incoordination. Because alcohol is almost instantaneously absorbed, those symptoms will show up within sixty minutes. You're home free if an hour passes without problems. If symptoms *do* occur, go to the emergency room.

A perfume or cologne splash to the eyes causes excruciating

iece of a mothball, for exam-
e a problem, because NPT dam-
d cells. On the other hand, even
DB crystals will cause little

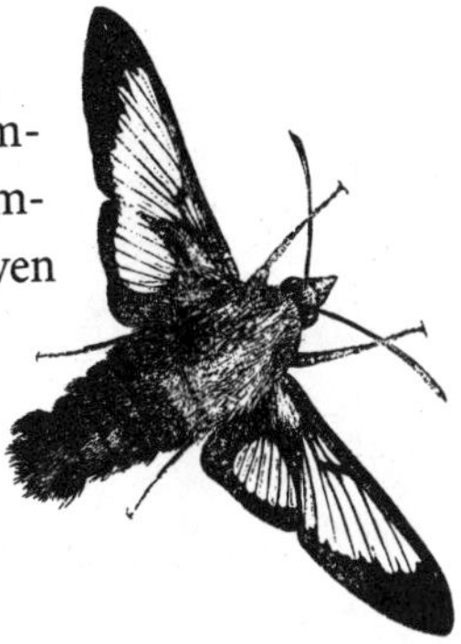

nothball ingestion, follow
nter's instructions. Don't use
s instructed to do so.

t

thalene is even more toxic in children born with an en-
ciency known as G6PD.
home remedy to repel animals in the attic is to spread
halene mothballs. However, as these mothballs evapo-
give off naphthalene fumes which, when inhaled, are
irritating and may even be dangerous. Never carelessly
othballs in an attic. If you must use them, leave them in
box in case they need to be removed. And by the way,
mals—like raccoons—won't be repelled by mothballs.
hey'll play with them.
main difference in the efficacy between naphthalene
dichlorobenzene is duration of action. Naphthalene
s last longer.

Bedroom

anufacturers are smart enough to realize that babies put
everything in their mouths. Accordingly, products made
are almost always nontoxic. That includes disposable di-
ugh a baby could choke on a piece); teething rings (usu-

pain, thanks to the alcohol. Alcohol irritates the eyes but won't harm them, so just rinse them for fifteen minutes with lukewarm water. Once you finish, the eyes will appear bloodshot and damaged. They're not. Give them about forty-five minutes to relax and they should start looking clear and normal. If they don't, see a doctor.

It's a Fact

- Hair sprays also contain alcohol, and while it's difficult to ingest enough hair spray to cause a problem, it's easy to spray one in the eyes. Follow the same treatment recommendations as for perfumes and colognes.
- Keep perfumed powders away from children. They may contain talc, which, when ingested, can get into the lungs and set up a form of pneumonia. If a talc ingestion occurs and persistent coughing, wheezing, or a fever develops later, seek medical help.

Softening the Skin

In general, any mild emollient cream or lotion—that is, one used to soften the skin—is minimally toxic. The only possible side effect is diarrhea if enough is ingested, owing to the oiliness of these products.

It's a Fact

- Lanolin is sometimes called "wool alcohol." However, despite the toxicological implications of that name, lanolin is nonalcoholic and nontoxic.
- Any petroleum jelly product—Vaseline, for example—can cause diarrhea when ingested but is considered nontoxic.
- Cold cream got its name because, as the water in the product evaporates, the skin feels cool. It's nontoxic.

Pregnancy Prevention Products and Sexual Aids

Sperm aren't very durable. All it takes to knock them out is a form of soap called nonoxynol 9. You'll find nonox in almost every spermicidal ointment, gel, or foam, and if some is ingested you might see mild vomiting. Give a glass of fluid.

Diarrhea might occur from eating a lubricant jelly—K-Y, for example. But these products are, like petroleum jelly, nontoxic. (Condom makers will tell you, however, that they're *not* exactly like petroleum jelly, and one should not replace the other as a lubricant.)

Speaking of condoms, they should be kept out of a child's reach for more than reasons of embarassment. A swallowed condom can prove a deadly obstruction in the throat. A *used* condom is no more or less poisonous than a fresh one, unless one of the adults has a sexually transmitted disease. Semen itself is nontoxic.

Men who use nonprescription ointments to sustain erections, take note: Some of these contain benzocaine, an anesthetic chemical that even in a small amount can cause a serious blood disorder in children called methemoglobinemia. Guys, hide these products somewhere with the condoms.

And while we're wrapping up the topic of sex, what about waterbed conditioners? Usually, these are made up of soap and water in a concentration that shouldn't cause any harm if swallowed. Dilute with a glass of fluid. You might see some vomiting.

Closet Talk

Silica Gel

Ever seen those little drums or packets inside of shoes, the ones imprinted with a skull and crossbones and a DO NOT EAT label? Well, you can eat all you want of what's inside these drums and it

will have no effect what
ent inside these package
ture to keep the shoes fr
We live in a litigious s
ing themselves against cl
or packets *could* be a cho
silica gel inside is inert; it
ing any effect.

Shoe Polish

Many shoe polishes als
of waxes and fats. But chec
ter, as some contain hydro
lowed might cause chemic
type you have, don't induc
gestion.
One extremely danger
sprays meant to protect lea
dirty. These repellents usu
when inhaled, cause dizzine
a coma if enough is inhaled.
products indoors. Take the sh

Mothballs

With the purchase of mot
to avoid a serious poisoning.
one far more poisonous than
are made of paradichlorobe
contain naphthalene (NPT).
children in the house. They'r
PDB.
Poison centers have varyin
toxic mothball exposure, but su

of NPT—a
ple—might b
ages red blo
one or two
harm.
For any
the poison c
ipecac unles

It's a Fa

• Naph
zyme def
• One
out naph
rate they
extremel
spread m
the open
some an
Instead,
• The
and para
mothbal

Baby's

Most
just about
for babies
apers (th

ally filled with either water or a glycerin-water mixture); and baby wipes (though there's a small amount of alcohol in some brands).

Infant Formula

One mistake new parents commonly make is in the mixing of infant formula. Unless you get it just right, the formula will be too strong for the baby's system to handle or won't contain enough nutrients to keep him growing.

For too-concentrated mixtures, diarrhea is the main threat. Usually, infants do just fine if you slightly increase their water intake. Too-dilute mixtures are less of an acute problem—the baby will usually just be hungry. But before embarking on any kind of fluid therapy with an infant, contact the pediatrician. Babies are highly sensitive to the amount of fluid they're getting.

It's a Fact

- Even though some infant formulas contain iron, it's unlikely a baby could develop iron poisoning from overconcentrated mixtures. There's just too little of the mineral there.

The Home Office

My, how the home office has changed! Twenty years ago, it consisted of a typewriter, correction fluid, and lots of pens and markers. Today it's a computer system where nothing gets printed until it's perfect on the screen. And when it gets printed, it's with some very toxic ink. The ink used in laser and ink-jet printers contains a high concentration of glycols. Glycols, as you may remember from the section on antifreeze, can cause kidney damage and raise the acidity of the blood.

But two things stand in the way of a poisoning from printer ink: the amount of ink contained in the printer cartridge and the cartridges themselves. They're small, difficult to get to, and hard to open. It's no surprise, then, that poison centers get few calls on computer ink ingestions.

Toner

If you're lucky enough to have a home copying machine, you're familiar with toner. The toxicity of toner really depends on the brand you use. Some toners—like Xerox—are mainly nontoxic. Others might cause minor symptoms if ingested. The best advice is to check with the poison center on the brand you use.

Pens and Markers

With pens and markers, you're dealing with highly toxic products that almost never cause a poisoning. There's just not enough ink to give us trouble, and what ink there is, is difficult to get to. So, for ink or Magic Marker "suckings," wipe out the mouth as best you can with a clean, wet cloth. If any unusual drowsiness seems to develop during the hour following the ink ingestion, go to the emergency room. But don't go crazy looking for it. It will almost never happen.

> **It's a Fact**
>
> • Bette Clair McMurray probably had no idea she was on the path to becoming a multimillionaire when she started bringing white paint to her job as a secretary to correct typing mistakes. But by 1959, she was filling orders out of her home for a hundred bottles a month of Liquid Paper. Twenty years later, her company was sold to Gillette for almost $150 million. McMurray's son, by the way, is Michael Nesmith, the former Monkee.

Correction Fluid

Finally, there's still room on the desk for that old correction fluid, only these days you can buy it in a water- or solvent-based formula. Opt for the water-based product, it's less toxic. The solvent-based formula contains trichloroethane, a compound related to chloroform. When inhaled, TCE causes dizziness and sleepiness. Again, be-

pain, thanks to the alcohol. Alcohol irritates the eyes but won't harm them, so just rinse them for fifteen minutes with lukewarm water. Once you finish, the eyes will appear bloodshot and damaged. They're not. Give them about forty-five minutes to relax and they should start looking clear and normal. If they don't, see a doctor.

It's a Fact

- Hair sprays also contain alcohol, and while it's difficult to ingest enough hair spray to cause a problem, it's easy to spray one in the eyes. Follow the same treatment recommendations as for perfumes and colognes.
- Keep perfumed powders away from children. They may contain talc, which, when ingested, can get into the lungs and set up a form of pneumonia. If a talc ingestion occurs and persistent coughing, wheezing, or a fever develops later, seek medical help.

Softening the Skin

In general, any mild emollient cream or lotion—that is, one used to soften the skin—is minimally toxic. The only possible side effect is diarrhea if enough is ingested, owing to the oiliness of these products.

It's a Fact

- Lanolin is sometimes called "wool alcohol." However, despite the toxicological implications of that name, lanolin is nonalcoholic and nontoxic.
- Any petroleum jelly product—Vaseline, for example—can cause diarrhea when ingested but is considered nontoxic.
- Cold cream got its name because, as the water in the product evaporates, the skin feels cool. It's nontoxic.

Pregnancy Prevention Products and Sexual Aids

Sperm aren't very durable. All it takes to knock them out is a form of soap called nonoxynol 9. You'll find nonox in almost every spermicidal ointment, gel, or foam, and if some is ingested you might see mild vomiting. Give a glass of fluid.

Diarrhea might occur from eating a lubricant jelly—K-Y, for example. But these products are, like petroleum jelly, nontoxic. (Condom makers will tell you, however, that they're *not* exactly like petroleum jelly, and one should not replace the other as a lubricant.)

Speaking of condoms, they should be kept out of a child's reach for more than reasons of embarassment. A swallowed condom can prove a deadly obstruction in the throat. A *used* condom is no more or less poisonous than a fresh one, unless one of the adults has a sexually transmitted disease. Semen itself is nontoxic.

Men who use nonprescription ointments to sustain erections, take note: Some of these contain benzocaine, an anesthetic chemical that even in a small amount can cause a serious blood disorder in children called methemoglobinemia. Guys, hide these products somewhere with the condoms.

And while we're wrapping up the topic of sex, what about waterbed conditioners? Usually, these are made up of soap and water in a concentration that shouldn't cause any harm if swallowed. Dilute with a glass of fluid. You might see some vomiting.

Closet Talk

Silica Gel

Ever seen those little drums or packets inside of shoes, the ones imprinted with a skull and crossbones and a DO NOT EAT label? Well, you can eat all you want of what's inside these drums and it will have no effect whatsoever. The highly nonpoisonous ingredient inside these packages is silica gel, a product that absorbs moisture to keep the shoes from getting destroyed by humidity.

We live in a litigious society, so the manufacturers are protecting themselves against claims they didn't warn you that the drums or packets *could* be a choking hazard if swallowed whole. But the silica gel inside is inert; it passes through the system without having any effect.

Shoe Polish

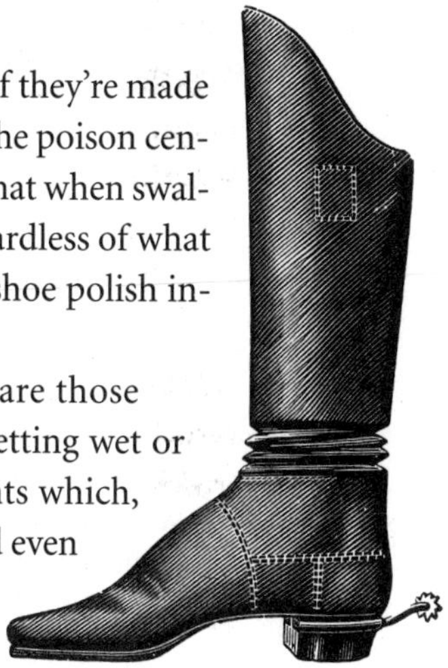

Many shoe polishes also have low toxicity, if they're made of waxes and fats. But check your brand with the poison center, as some contain hydrocarbons, materials that when swallowed might cause chemical pneumonia. Regardless of what type you have, don't induce vomiting with a shoe polish ingestion.

One extremely dangerous shoe product are those sprays meant to protect leather boots from getting wet or dirty. These repellents usually contain solvents which, when inhaled, cause dizziness, drowsiness, and even a coma if enough is inhaled. *Never spray these products indoors.* Take the shoes outside.

Mothballs

With the purchase of mothballs, you have a clear opportunity to avoid a serious poisoning. These products come in two types, one far more poisonous than the other. Less toxic moth crystals are made of paradichlorobenzene (PDB). The more toxic balls contain naphthalene (NPT). Avoid NPT mothballs if you've got children in the house. They're about six times more toxic than PDB.

Poison centers have varying standards for what constitutes a toxic mothball exposure, but suffice to say that even small amounts

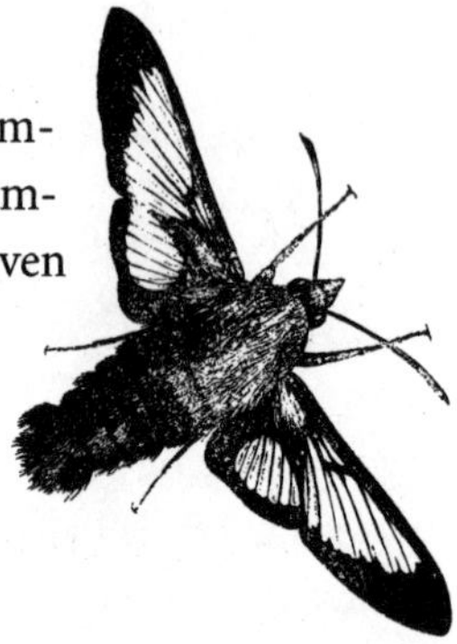

of NPT—a piece of a mothball, for example—might be a problem, because NPT damages red blood cells. On the other hand, even one or two PDB crystals will cause little harm.

For any mothball ingestion, follow the poison center's instructions. Don't use ipecac unless instructed to do so.

It's a Fact

• Naphthalene is even more toxic in children born with an enzyme deficiency known as G6PD.

• One home remedy to repel animals in the attic is to spread out naphthalene mothballs. However, as these mothballs evaporate they give off naphthalene fumes which, when inhaled, are extremely irritating and may even be dangerous. Never carelessly spread mothballs in an attic. If you must use them, leave them in the open box in case they need to be removed. And by the way, some animals—like raccoons—won't be repelled by mothballs. Instead, they'll play with them.

• The main difference in the efficacy between naphthalene and paradichlorobenzene is duration of action. Naphthalene mothballs last longer.

Baby's Bedroom

Most manufacturers are smart enough to realize that babies put just about everything in their mouths. Accordingly, products made for babies are almost always nontoxic. That includes disposable diapers (though a baby could choke on a piece); teething rings (usually filled with either water or a glycerin-water mixture); and baby wipes (though there's a small amount of alcohol in some brands).

Infant Formula

One mistake new parents commonly make is in the mixing of infant formula. Unless you get it just right, the formula will be too strong for the baby's system to handle or won't contain enough nutrients to keep him growing.

For too-concentrated mixtures, diarrhea is the main threat. Usually, infants do just fine if you slightly increase their water intake. Too-dilute mixtures are less of an acute problem—the baby will usually just be hungry. But before embarking on any kind of fluid therapy with an infant, contact the pediatrician. Babies are highly sensitive to the amount of fluid they're getting.

It's a Fact

- Even though some infant formulas contain iron, it's unlikely a baby could develop iron poisoning from overconcentrated mixtures. There's just too little of the mineral there.

The Home Office

My, how the home office has changed! Twenty years ago, it consisted of a typewriter, correction fluid, and lots of pens and markers. Today it's a computer system where nothing gets printed until it's perfect on the screen. And when it gets printed, it's with some very toxic ink. The ink used in laser and ink-jet printers contains a high concentration of glycols. Glycols, as you may remember from the section on antifreeze, can cause kidney damage and raise the acidity of the blood.

But two things stand in the way of a poisoning from printer ink: the amount of ink contained in the printer cartridge and the cartridges themselves. They're small, difficult to get to, and hard to open. It's no surprise, then, that poison centers get few calls on computer ink ingestions.

Toner

If you're lucky enough to have a home copying machine, you're familiar with toner. The toxicity of toner really depends on the brand you use. Some toners—like Xerox—are mainly nontoxic. Others might cause minor symptoms if ingested. The best advice is to check with the poison center on the brand you use.

Pens and Markers

With pens and markers, you're dealing with highly toxic products that almost never cause a poisoning. There's just not enough ink to give us trouble, and what ink there is, is difficult to get to. So, for ink or Magic Marker "suckings," wipe out the mouth as best you can with a clean, wet cloth. If any unusual drowsiness seems to develop during the hour following the ink ingestion, go to the emergency room. But don't go crazy looking for it. It will almost never happen.

Correction Fluid

Finally, there's still room on the desk for that old correction fluid, only these days you can buy it in a water- or solvent-based formula. Opt for the water-based product, it's less toxic. The solvent-based formula contains trichloroethane, a compound related to chloroform. When inhaled, TCE causes dizziness and sleepiness. Again, be-

It's a Fact

- Bette Clair McMurray probably had no idea she was on the path to becoming a multimillionaire when she started bringing white paint to her job as a secretary to correct typing mistakes. But by 1959, she was filling orders out of her home for a hundred bottles a month of Liquid Paper. Twenty years later, her company was sold to Gillette for almost $150 million. McMurray's son, by the way, is Michael Nesmith, the former Monkee.

cause of the way in which it's packaged you're unlikely to see an inhalation problem with correction fluid, unless—it happens—there's a thrill seeker in the house trying to get high by intentionally inhaling the stuff. For an ingestion of the water-based formula—and it's bound to be a small ingestion because of the way it's packaged—rinse out the mouth. For the solvent-based formula, do the same but also observe for about an hour for drowsiness. If it occurs, go to the emergency room.

8

The Living Room and the Family Room

Here's the room where we indulge many of our worst personal habits—especially drinking and smoking. The problem is, we sometimes leave remnants of those habits behind when we head up to bed, such that children can partake of our addictions the next day by, for example, chewing down a cigarette butt or drinking the remainder of an alcoholic drink. Be especially vigilant about keeping tobacco products—*all* tobacco products—away from children. And if you're trying to kick the habit with the aid of some of that Nicorette gum, more power to you. But keep in mind it's highly toxic as well.

Nicotine

Nicotine is one of the most dangerous substances found in the home. We're not just talking about its long-term effects on the heart and lungs, but about the danger to children from acute nicotine poisoning, such as you might find when a child ingests a cigarette, cigar, chewing tobacco, or even a nicotine gum meant to prevent smoking.

There's lots of danger down tobacco road. The stomach hates nicotine and reacts with revulsion when a tobacco product is swallowed. Vomiting is the usual result. The intestines feel the same way. In fact, smoking can stimulate a bowel movement. In children, that can mean diarrhea. But it's the cardiovascular system that takes the biggest hit from nicotine: The heart rate increases and the blood pressure soars following use of the drug. In a worst-case scenario, that could result in a stroke.

In terms of nicotine concentration, the most dangerous form of tobacco is snuff—tobacco that's stuffed up the nostrils. Some brands of snuff contain so much nicotine that it would take just half a teaspoonful to kill a child.

Chewing tobacco, sometimes called "chaw," is stuck between the gum and lip, and the user frequently spits out pieces of chaw and wads of tainted saliva. If that isn't stomach-turning enough, how about this: Children sometimes drink this chaw-tainted saliva. Because we can't tell precisely what the concentration of the nicotine is in a given sample of spittle, any chaw or chaw/saliva ingestion should be treated as an emergency.

For cigarettes, we can define an amount that might be toxic, but consult your local poison center for its parameters. Ingesting a smallish piece of a cigarette or cigar, or a couple of cigarette butts, can usually be handled at home. Vomiting is likely. If the vomiting is severe, go to the emergency room. If it's minor, treat at home by replenishing fluids, ideally with sips of an electrolyte drink like Pedialyte.

Chewing on a cigar without swallowing any of it may cause vomiting as well. When you call the

It's a Fact

- Some cigarettes contain less nicotine than others, but no cigarette is nontoxic.
- Pipe tobacco is also highly toxic.
- Since 1859, matches have been made of the same material: potassium chlorate. You'd have to eat at least a book of matches to get a toxic exposure.
- And while we're on the subject of ashes, fireplace residues are usually nontoxic. However, partially burned chunks can get stuck in the throat. Also, never burn pressure-treated wood in the fireplace. It contains highly poisonous chemicals—arsenic, for one.

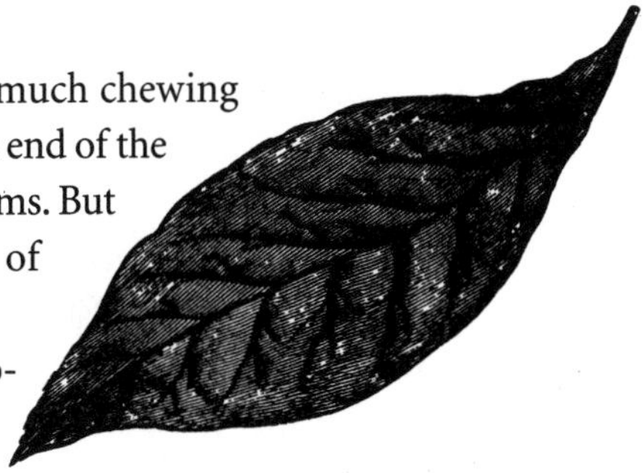

poison center, try to quantify how much chewing has been done. A simple chew on the end of the cigar is not likely to result in symptoms. But chomping on a stogie in imitation of Grandpa might be a problem.

Perhaps the most dangerous nicotine product is Nicorette gum, available over the counter—not so much because it contains loads of nicotine, as because all gum is attractive to children. Just one block of Nicorette, chewed by a child, could result in nausea, vomiting, and even some dangerous cardiac symptoms. *Nicorette is a dangerous product. In a home where there are children, be extremely careful where you store it.* Also, be sure to dispose of chewed-up pieces of Nicorette where children and pets can't get to them. Used Nicorette pieces can contain substantial quantities of nicotine. Nicotine patches, also now available over the counter, aren't as appetizing as Nicorette gum, but if chewed they too can be toxic.

Living Room Appliances

Among the items sold for VCR maintenance is the tape head cleaner, meant to be used every once in a while to keep the player free of dust and grit. Usually, tape head cleaners contain nothing more than isopropyl—rubbing—alcohol. A small taste of a tape head cleaner won't cause a problem. Give a glass of juice. A substantial ingestion—and it's hard to imagine someone enjoying a tape head cleaner enough to make a cocktail out of it—merits an emergency room visit, especially if we're talking about a child. Isopropyl alcohol severely irritates the stomach and induces deep drowsiness.

The only other living room appliance of note is the air conditioner. As with the refrigerator, a freon leak can sometimes occur as the coils of the air conditioning unit age or if they are mistakenly pierced. Freon smells like a newly cut lawn, but you may not smell anything. Instead, coughing and other minor respiratory systems will ensue. A freon leak from a home air conditioner is normally not dangerous. Unplug the unit and keep the windows open until it can be repaired. And yes, it can be left overnight, provided there's enough ventilation in the room.

It's a Fact

• Anyone who suffers from cardiac arrhythmias is at higher risk from a freon leak than a healthy person, as freon sensitizes the heart, sometimes causing it to beat irregularly.

• Willis H. Carrier is considered the father of air-conditioning.

• Early air conditioners (c. 1920) used ammonia. Freon was discovered in 1930.

Furniture and Upholstery Cleaners

Oils and Polishes

By and large, furniture oils and polishes contain hydrocarbons, those petroleum products that, if ingested, can get into the lungs and cause pneumonia. So don't induce vomiting after a furniture polish ingestion. Instead, observe for six hours. If coughing, wheezing, or fever develop, go to the emergency room. "Oil soaps" may contain no oils at all. For example, Murphy's Oil Soap is made up of low-toxicity detergents and water.

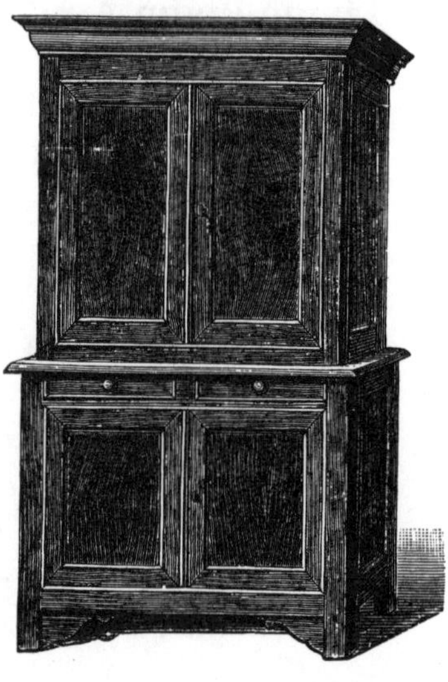

Upholstery Cleaners

Generally low in toxicity, home upholstery cleaners contain various soaps and solvents. An ingestion might cause an upset stomach and even some vomiting, but it shouldn't be severe. Give a glass of fluid and observe. You're highly unlikely to see a problem with a home rug cleaner either. They, too, are usually made up of soaps. Hardwood floor cleaners might contain some toxic glycol compounds, but probably in a low concentration. A taste should be no problem.

It's a Fact

- Vacuum cleaner tablets are normally nontoxic.
- Rug and upholstery deodorizers usually contain odor-absorbing sodium bicarbonate—baking soda. Sodium bicarbonate is only poisonous if a large amount is ingested.
- Many upholstery and rug cleaners contain glycol solvents. Theoretically, these should be extremely toxic, but practically speaking they don't seem to be.

The Liquor Cabinet

One Christmas Eve, a couple made a mistake. Instead of feeding their baby milk from the refrigerator, they fed him Kahlúa and milk already mixed for a party. The baby enjoyed the drink heartily but wound up in the emergency room with alcohol poisoning.

Children should not be fed alcohol. Alcohol affects kids more drastically than adults. It causes a quick drop in blood sugar, drowsiness, and even coma. Certainly, a sip of alcohol is not likely to result in terrible symptoms. But alcohol poisoning is dependent on weight. The smaller the child, the less alcohol the child can tolerate. Notify the poison center of any alcohol ingestion by a child.

9

The Toy Box and Unusual Poisons

With children, nothing's out of the realm of possibility when it comes to an ingestion. In this chapter we look at some of the strange things kids get into and some common toys that often wind up in their mouths, plus a look at holiday hazards, those once-a-year possibilities for a poisoning.

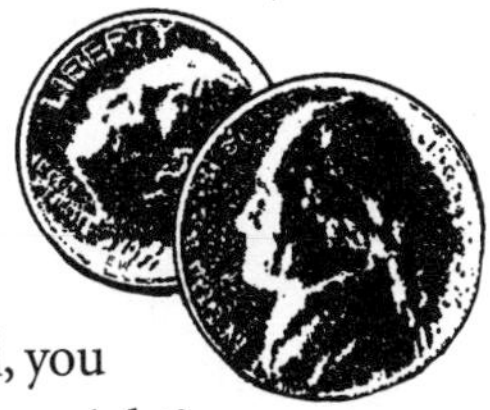

Odd Problems

Small Change

Your two-year-old son swallows a coin. No big deal, you think. He isn't choking, so there couldn't be a problem, right?

Perhaps. You *might* be right—the coin could've passed right down to his stomach where, in a few days, it will come out through the anus. But there's something about the shape of a coin that sometimes allows it to get stuck in the throat without any symptoms of choking. In fact, there is at least one undocumented case I know of where a coin was stuck in the throat for so long that the body began to grow tissue around it.

The trouble with coins stuck in the throat is that sooner or later they become unstuck. It might happen a few minutes after the ingestion, or a few hours. But whenever it becomes dislodged, there's a fresh opportunity for choking. So if your child swallows a coin, do nothing yourself but get the child to the emergency room. They'll X-ray the throat and abdomen to pinpoint the location of the coin. If it's stuck in the throat, an endoscope can be passed down to remove it. If it's in the stomach there's no immediate problem, and the hospital will usually arrange for a follow-up X ray to make sure it has passed through the bowels. (You'll also be asked to watch for the coin in the feces.)

It's a Fact

• While all coin ingestions are potentially dangerous, the worst ones are dimes and pennies because they're easily swallowed. Thicker and larger nickels and quarters are more likely to cause immediate choking.

• The metals that make up coins are usually of no toxic consequence with an ingestion.

• Any coin-shaped object—washers, tokens, etc.—can also become stuck in the throat, so keep these away from children, as well.

Batteries

Tiny watch and hearing-aid batteries, on the other hand, usually don't cause choking. Instead, they slide on down to the stomach, where they can dissolve and cause a burn. These batteries contain corrosive materials, and it's imperative that they pass through the system without dissolving. Take a child who has ingested a battery to the emergency room.

The first step is to find where the battery has settled via an X ray. Batteries that have crept into the distant reaches of the stomach are best left to pass through the system on their own. Those in the upper part of the stomach can be retrieved using an endoscope. Usually it takes three to five days for a battery to pass through the intestines, and a follow-up X ray is done around that time. Batteries that remain stuck in the intestines may have to be dislodged using laxatives.

Larger batteries—the kind that go in transistor radios or tiny flashlights—are usually too large to be swallowed without choking. But anything's possible. And if one of these manages to make its way to the stomach, there could be severe damage if it leaks. Report to the emergency room if one of these has been swallowed.

As batteries age, they sometimes leak the corrosive material potassium hydroxide. Licking an intact battery isn't toxic, but licking the ooze from a leaking battery can burn the mouth. Look for blisters, peeling skin, or other signs of a burn in the mouth or on the lips. If you see any of these signs see a doctor. If you don't, keep it in the back of your mind that any difficulty in swallowing or speaking or any excessive drooling that develops later in the day might be due to a throat burn. Seek medical attention if any of these things occur.

Photographs

If you've got a darkroom at home, you probably know the chemicals used to develop film are quite toxic. But the photographs themselves, when dry, are not toxic when chewed.

Products for Animals

Cat litter, when clean, is nontoxic—unless someone sits down and makes a meal out of it. With large amounts, the relatively small amount of fluid in the body's stomach and intestines will cause the clay that comprises cat litter to swell. That could cause a blockage. So, after any cat litter ingestion—and it's likely to be a small one—give a good-sized glass of water or juice. Any persistent stomach cramping, especially if accompanied by constipation, might indicate more cat litter was eaten than you think. But frankly, it's hard to believe that could happen.

Remember the stories about elderly people eating cat food instead of tuna fish? Well, none of them died as a result. Cat and dog food might be disgusting, but they're not toxic. Same goes for fish food.

Animal feces, on the other hand, could be a problem. The issue is parasites. Even domestic animals—especially cats—can harbor dangerous parasites. An ingestion of animal feces could result in a severe, even fatal infection.

Cats carry toxoplasmosis, a parasite that's especially harmful to the developing fetus. Pregnant women should never clean out cat litter boxes and should, in fact, stay away from cats. Children who ingest cat feces may need to have the stomach emptied using ipecac syrup. Check with your poison center. The same is generally true of feces from other animals.

Urine

An unusual set of circumstances would need to converge to cause a dangerous ingestion of urine.

Because urine is sterile when it leaves the body, it's not intrinsically harmful if ingested. It's possible that urine can contain bacteria if a person has a urinary tract infection. In that case, ingesting urine might be like ingesting contaminated food—depending on the bacteria we're talking about, of course. That might result in nausea, vomiting, and diarrhea.

But that's an extremely unlikely scenario, so for all intents and purposes, an ingestion of human urine should be considered nontoxic. The only realistic exposure to animal urine might be from ingesting contaminated cat litter. Again, the urine itself would probably not be toxic, but because the cat normally sits to urinate, its anus—which *could* be contaminated with parasites—might deposit these bugs on the cat litter. The bottom line: Never let small children play with or around a cat litter box.

Toys and Hobby Materials

Super Glue

No doubt, some of the more amusing calls to poison centers result from Super Glue exposures like these: a woman who glued her head to a lamp while watching *Sesame Street;* a two-year-old who glued her vagina shut; a man who glued his hand to his glasses, and another who glued his hand to his penis.

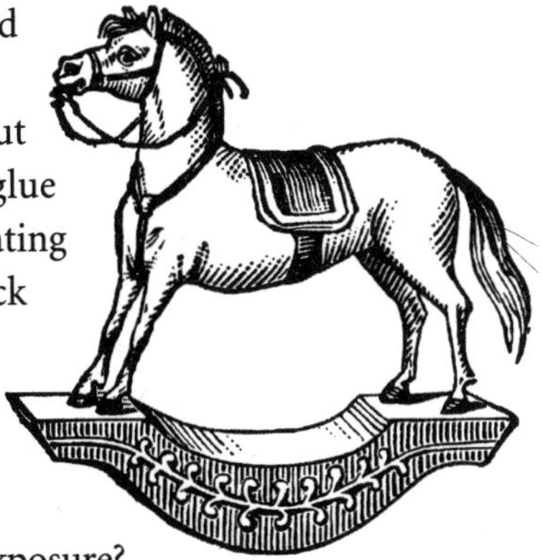

Powerful stuff, that Super Glue, but minimally toxic. Super Glue, or any glue made from a cyanoacrylate, isn't irritating or harmful if ingested. But it will stick things together so that they can't be torn apart. And when skin is involved, you shouldn't *try* to pull things apart, or you might rip the skin off.

So what to do about a Super Glue exposure? That depends on what body part we're talking about. For most adhesions, simply soak the affected area in warm water for thirty to sixty minutes and then use vegetable oil or petroleum jelly to ease the tissues apart.

Swallowing Super Glue isn't harmful. In fact, it hardens so fast there's almost no chance it will get past the tonsils as a liquid. It might stick to the teeth and tongue, but it's perfectly safe to let it wear off on its own. Or, if it's really bothering you, use a *soft* toothbrush and gently run it over the teeth and gums. If you encounter resistance, leave it alone.

Some poison centers recommend that Super Glue in the eyes is best handled in the emergency room. But many times an "eye" exposure of Super Glue doesn't involve the eyes at all but the eyelids. For eyelid exposures, apply a warm compress to the area for thirty to sixty minutes. *Never forcibly pull apart the eyelids.* The tissue is thin and can tear, so if you encounter any resistance, seek medical help. And obviously, if the eyes *are* involved seek medical help before doing anything.

Other Glues

That kindergarten companion Elmer's glue is nontoxic and easily removed from the skin with soap and water. Model cements, brush cleaners, and thinners used for plastic and wood models often contain highly toxic, aromatic materials like xylene. These products should never be used by young children and never without ventilation for everyone else, as they cause dizziness and drowsiness when inhaled. If this happens, get fresh air. Minor symptoms should resolve quickly. Never induce vomiting for an ingestion of a model glue product that contains xylene. Drowsiness could quickly ensue, and some of these glues also contain hydrocarbons that can cause chemical pneumonia if they're inhaled.

Testor's, a big player in the model cement business, has available a nontoxic glue for younger children to use.

Paints and Crayons

Fingerpaints, watercolor sets, crayons, chalk, and children's felt-tip pens are generally nontoxic. But beware products made by unknown firms from other countries. A few years ago, some imported crayons were found to contain lead.

Paints made for dressing up plastic and wood models *can* be toxic. But they come in such small inaccessible bottles that poisonings are rare.

Chemistry Sets

Toy chemistry sets usually contain minimally toxic ingredients. Some of these have laxative properties (phenolphthalein, guar gum); some upset the stomach (borax). But most ingredients are safe *for older children.* The last thing toymakers need is a slew of lawsuits over a chemistry set, so they've got a strong incentive to keep things low in toxicity. Still, chemistry set items should never be eaten, as some side effects are possible.

Fuels for Toys

Be extremely careful with the fuel used to power toy planes, boats, and cars. Some of these contain the deadly ingredients nitroethane and methanol. If ingested, nitroethane can cause methemoglobinemia, a severe blood disorder, while methanol can cause

It's a Fact

- Lead pencils don't contain lead. They contain nontoxic graphite. Pencil erasers are also nontoxic.
- Don't worry about a leaking toy baby bottle. The liquid inside is nontoxic.
- The liquid that makes toy train engines "smoke" is usually just mineral oil. It could cause pneumonia if it got into the lungs, but it's mainly a laxative.
- Play-Doh contains nothing toxic, but it's not food and shouldn't be eaten; ditto for Silly Putty.
- Glowing nightsticks are known in the poison center trade as Cyalumes. These contain a liquid ingredient called dibutyl phthalate that's pretty much nontoxic. However, Cyalume fluid splashed into the eyes will sting. Treat it at home with a fifteen-minute lukewarm water flush.
- More nontoxic toys: GAK, SMUD, and FLOAM.
- Most Tinker Bell toy cosmetic products are nontoxic. But at least one brand of toy nail polish contains the eye irritant dibutyl phthalate. Some toy body powders contains the lung irritant talc, and some toy perfumes contain alcohol. Nonalcohol toy perfumes contain the relatively nontoxic propylene glycol.
- Magic Rocks, a set of crystals to grow rocks, are made of sodium silicate, which can be very irritating—even corrosive—if swallowed or splashed into the eyes.
- Solutions for blowing bubbles are essentially liquid soaps. They're not especially toxic but can cause diarrhea if ingested.

blindness. *Always consider ingestions of model fuels an emergency.* Don't induce vomiting. Call the poison center and be prepared to head to a hospital. Eye exposures, on the other hand, can be handled at home with a fifteen-minute lukewarm water rinse. Never let a methanol-containing product sit on the skin, as the toxin can be absorbed.

Holiday Hazards

Valentine's Day

As they say in the toxins trade, poisonings never take a holiday. Even Valentine's Day presents a hazard—for dogs. Chocolate speeds up a dog's heart rate so much it can send the animal into cardiac arrest. A piece or two of chocolate won't do it, but dogs who tear open candy boxes and eat everything inside might need to see a vet. It really depends on the dog's weight.

Easter

A month or so later, it's Easter egg–coloring time. The tablets contain nontoxic food dyes, baking soda, and/or sodium chloride—table salt. It's doubtful you'll see any kind of a large ingestion with these, as they taste awful. And a few tablets aren't likely to cause any harm. But because salt and baking soda are involved, toxicity will depend on the child's weight.

It's a Fact

- Hard-boiled eggs decorated for Easter should be kept refrigerated if you plan to eat them. It's okay to take them out for a short Easter egg hunt, but return them to cold storage as soon as possible; otherwise you're risking food poisoning.

Halloween

Some Halloween parties feature a big bowl of punch with smoke rising from the top. Dry ice makes this vaporous effect possible. Dry ice, which is really just frozen carbon dioxide, is nontoxic. But don't try to eat it or you might get frostbite inside your mouth. Don't handle dry ice without gloves, either.

The severity of a dry ice burn will depend on duration of contact. Some are minor; some result in deep destruction of tissue. Your objective in treating a dry ice burn is to warm the tissue without further damaging it. So gradual warming is a better idea than, say, sticking the affected part in a flame. Warm water is one option. Any area that remains white and without feeling needs to be treated by a doctor.

Christmas

Along with the gifts, cookies, and candy, we introduce a number of poisonous plants and objects into our homes at Christmas. Let us first dispel a monstrous myth about one Christmas plant: *Poinsettias are not poisonous.* They may look like the death stars of Christmas, with their brilliant red color, but it would take a wheelbarrowful of poinsettia leaves to cause a problem—and the problem would probably be nothing more than a bad stomachache. So don't worry about poinsettia plants. A related species also seen around Christmas is the crown of thorns plant. Ingestions may cause vomiting, and the sap is irritating to the eyes and skin, but again, it's not extremely toxic.

Do worry about mistletoe, but not overly so. Eating a few mistletoe berries might cause an upset stomach, but it's the rest of the plant that's more toxic. It's possible that an ingestion of mistletoe, if large enough (and that's an inexact number), could cause the blood pressure to climb and seizures to occur. So even though a serious problem with mistletoe berries is unlikely, it's a good idea to use fake mistletoe in your foyer.

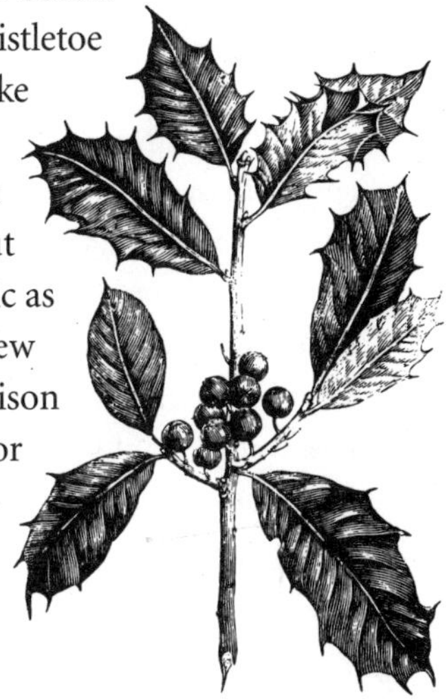

What would Christmas be without holly berries? A little safer, perhaps. But holly berries aren't anywhere near as toxic as folk tales would have you believe. A few berries might cause an upset stomach. Poison centers tend to have differing standards for what constitutes a toxic holly berry exposure, but suffice to say that fewer than five berries will probably not require treatment.

The Christmas tree itself isn't poisonous, but the sharp needles of pines can damage and become stuck in the throat. Call 911 if you see evidence of trouble talking, swallowing, or breathing following a pine needle exposure. It's the same story with artificial trees: They're not poisonous, but the plastic needles can be sharp. The powder you sprinkle into the tree stand to keep the tree fresh usually contains nothing more than sugar. It's not toxic.

Most Christmas tree decorations are nontoxic. The only things you really need to worry about are old ornaments—which might be decorated with lead paint—and anything else that could get stuck in a child's throat. It's best, really, to minimize your problems at Christmas. Keep the tree decorating simple: lights, ornaments, perhaps some nontoxic fake snow or a string of popcorn and cranberries. Children can choke on things like icicles and pieces of garland, so steer clear of them until they're older.

Take care, also, with house decorations—especially potpourris. By and large, potpourri ingestions are usually small and thus don't result in a serious problem. But the potential is there. Dry potpourris, which usually sit out in an open bowl, contain sharp objects that can damage the inside of the mouth and throat and possibly cause choking. Otherwise, they're low in toxicity. Potpourri oils, used in rings around lamps and in "simmering" potpourris, sometimes contain highly toxic essential oils. These oils are so concentrated that a small ingestion—even as little as a teaspoonful or two—can cause serious drowsiness, even a coma. But potpourris normally contain only a bit of these essential oils, so it's unlikely you'll see a problem with a small ingestion.

Finally, those little snow toys you shake up contain tiny particles of plastic. Plastic isn't toxic and the water inside *should* be okay, too. But it could contain bacteria. So if the water is ingested, observe for nausea, vomiting, or diarrhea. If they occur, see a doctor.

Part II

The Medicine Cabinet

Most home poisonings involve drugs, prescription and nonprescription. And in many cases, the first crucial element in determining toxicity is the weight-to-dose ratio: How much does the person weigh, and how much medicine was taken? Always have an updated idea of each family member's weight. That way, you'll avoid having to stumble around in a panic looking for a scale when a poisoning occurs.

Second, try to keep accurate track of how much medicine you've got in the house—even if it's only a rough idea. Many drug poisonings can be handled at home if a small amount has been ingested. The problem is, if you don't know how much of a drug you had in the first place, you can't accurately assess how much someone might've taken. Lack of information is almost always a straight path to the emergency room. So keep an inventory of drugs in and drugs out. And always dispose of drugs that are out of date or that you have finished using.

Third, never use ipecac syrup unless instructed to do so by a poison center. This rule applies to all home poisonings, but it's particularly important with drugs, because many cause drowsiness and seizures—not ideal conditions under which to be vomiting.

Fourth, remember that many highly toxic prescription drugs are found in the homes of grandparents. Know what *they're* taking, as well, and encourage them to adopt child-safe storage for their medications. As children get older, safe *storage* becomes a more important consideration than safety caps. *There is no such thing as a childproof cap.* Some are child-resistant, but that doesn't mean they can't be pried off. Your best bet is to put all medications under lock and key.

And finally, for every poisoning—but especially with drugs—it's important to call your local poison control center. Toxicology is a constantly evolving discipline. By contacting a poison center, you're not only getting the latest treatment information available, you're contributing to the data base information about how drugs affect the body in an overdose. Poison centers *need* that information to improve on the advice they give. So always call them when there's a poisoning.

10

Prescription Drugs

The drugs in this chapter appear under the conditions for which they are prescribed, which in turn are listed alphabetically, from *acne* to *viral infections.* Sections on discontinued medications and illicit drugs are also included.

Some drugs that recently hit the market aren't covered because they have no toxicological history—not enough people have been poisoned by them yet to give accurate advice on treatment. As for the rating scale you see in this chapter—**Probable toxicity**—it's based on two things: how intrinsically toxic the drug is and how involved the treatment of an overdose.

Acne

Tretinoin (Retin-A)

Probable toxicity: Low. Originally developed to treat acne, tretinoin seems to have found its niche not with teenagers but with aging baby boomers. Once word got out that tretinoin cream took out facial wrinkles, the drug really took off. At most, you might see an upset stomach with an ingestion of tretinoin cream.

Overdose recommendation: Call poison center.

Likely treatment: None.

It's a fact: You can thank University of Pennsylvania researcher Albert Kligman for tretinoin. Kligman discovered the drug some thirty years ago.

Isotretinoin (Accutane)

Probable toxicity: Low. Somewhat similar to vitamin A, isotretinoin capsules have little toxicity if accidentally ingested.

Overdose recommendation: Call poison center.

Likely treatment: None.

It's a fact: Accutane *is* highly toxic to the developing fetus. Pregnant women should never use Accutane.

Allergies

Astemizole (Hismanal), clemastine (Tavist), hydroxyzine (Vistaril), loratadine (Claritin), terfenadine (Seldane)

Probable toxicity: Low to moderate. These drugs counteract the effect of histamine, a chemical in the body that produces the symptoms you see in allergic reactions: itchy, watery eyes, wheezing, rash, and swelling. You will surely see side effects in an overdose, most probably drowsiness. However, small overdoses are generally mild and many times can be left untreated.

Overdose recommendation: No ipecac. Call poison center.

Likely treatment: None for a small overdose; gastric lavage and use of activated charcoal for a large one.

It's a fact: Some children who ingest antihistamines have what's called a "paradoxical reaction." Instead of getting sleepy they become hyperactive.

Anxiety and Sleep

Benzodiazepines: Alprazolam (Xanax), chlordiazepoxide (Librium), clorazepate (Tranxene), diazepam (Valium), estazolam (ProSom), flurazepam (Dalmane), halazepam (Paxipam), lorazepam (Ativan), oxazepam (Serax), prazepam (Centrax), quazepam (Doral); temazepam (Restoril), triazolam (Halcion), also zolpidem (Ambien)

Probable toxicity: Low to moderate. Librium, the first drug in this class, was discovered by accident back in the late 1950s. It was quickly followed into the marketplace by the legendary Valium. Despite the negative connotation now attached to Valium and the other drugs in this class, they are extremely safe. The fact is, even massive overdoses of a benzodiazepine—taken without any other drugs or alcohol—will cause sleepiness but not death. Just ask Bud McFarlane, President Reagan's former national security adviser, who attempted suicide during the Iran-Contra affair by taking an overdose of Valium. He survived. Throw in a few sips of whiskey with Valium, though, and all bets are off.

Overdose recommendation: No ipecac. Call poison center.

Likely treatment: For a tablet or two, home observation is usually all that's necessary. You'll be watching for excessive drowsiness. Alprazolam is sometimes treated as a more potent drug than the others, so even a small ingestion may be sent in to the hospital; the same is true for zolpidem. Severe overdoses might be treated with flumazenil, a drug that reverses benzodiazepine toxicity.

It's a fact: Bad press has followed Halcion for years. The drug has been banned in several European countries for being too powerful a sleep agent, and, like Prozac, it has been blamed for pushing a few individuals to commit homicide.

Other sedatives: Chloral hydrate (Noctec), dichloralphenazone (Midrin), ethchlorvynol (Placidyl)

Probable toxicity: High. Gradually, these older sedatives are being phased from use. However, chloral hydrate, one of the oldest drugs still in use (it was introduced in 1860), is often prescribed for children as a sedative, particularly before some diagnostic procedures. Dichloralphenazone, used in the migraine drug Midrin, breaks down to chloral hydrate when metabolized (Midrin also contains acetaminophen). Ethchlorvynol, rarely used anymore, is a minty-tasting, highly dangerous drug that produces comatose states of shocking duration; two weeks isn't unusual.

Overdose recommendation: No ipecac. Call poison center. Hospital visit probable.

Likely treatment: Treatment will consist of cleaning out the stomach, a dose of activated charcoal, and a long period of observation. Commonly, chloral hydrate upsets the stomach.

It's a fact: Chloral hydrate gained notoriety as an ingredient in the toxic drink Mickey Finn.

Meprobamate (Equanil, Miltown)

Probable toxicity: High. The granddaddy of the modern sedatives, meprobamate was introduced in 1955 as a drug that was "non–habit forming" and wouldn't dull or deaden the senses. But by 1963 one medical journal reported that an alarming number of suicidal ingestions were linked to meprobamate. It's been falling from favor for years, but you'll still find meprobamate in some homes.

Overdose recommendation: No ipecac. Call poison center.

Likely treatment: For children, meprobamate ingestions are best treated or observed in the emergency room. Big ingestors get gastric lavage and activated charcoal.

It's a fact: Felbamate (Felbatol), an antiseizure drug chemically related to meprobamate, had a short turbulent history in the marketplace. Introduced in 1993, felbamate was soon linked to potentially fatal blood and liver problems. It's now sold under strict controls.

Asthma

Mast cell stabilizers: Cromolyn sodium (Intal), nedocromil sodium (Tilade)

Probable toxicity: Low. At this point, the drug firm that introduced cromolyn more than twenty years ago for asthma has managed to get approval to stuff it into a number of bodily orifices, including orally, where it's used to treat mastocytosis, an allergic condition affecting the intestinal tract. The toxic effects of nedocromil are similarly low.

Overdose recommendation: Ingestions of cromolyn or nedocromil should result in no toxicity whatsoever.

Likely treatment: None.

It's a fact: These drugs prevent allergic reactions by preventing the release of histamine from "mast cells"—cells that burst open during an allergic reaction to release histamine and other chemicals that cause swelling, redness, and itching.

Xanthines: Aminophylline, oxtryphilline (Choledyl), theophylline (Slo-Bid, Slo-Phyllin, Theo-24, Theo-Dur); also contained in some nonprescription asthma medications like Tedral.

Probable toxicity: High. How does "coffee-ground" vomiting grab you? That's one of the unsavory side effects of a xanthine overdose—a blackish-colored vomit made up of partially digested blood cells. But xanthines don't just irritate the stomach, they make the heart pump so hard and so fast that cardiac arrest can occur. They also cause seizures.

Overdose recommendation: Call poison center. Dire as xanthine poisoning sounds, small overdoses can sometimes be treated at home.

Likely treatment: Could range from using syrup of ipecac at home to the works: pumping the stomach, admittance to the hospital with careful monitoring, even renal dialysis or a similar decontamination procedure called charcoal hemoperfusion, in which the blood is passed through a charcoal column.
It's a fact: Think of these drugs as molecules of supercharged caffeine, a chemical to which they're related. Even small overdoses can produce jitteriness and a quickened heartbeat.

Inhalers containing steroids: Beclomethasone (Beclovent, Vanceril), budesonide (Rhinocort), dexamethasone (Dexacort), flunisolide (Aerobid), triamcinolone (Azmacort)

Probable toxicity: Low to moderate. Acute overuse of these drugs is not a problem. Long-term high-dose use affects the function of the adrenal glands.

Overdose recommendation: No ipecac. Call poison center.

Likely treatment: None in most cases.

It's a fact: Aerosol inhalant abuse can sometimes be deadly, not necessarily owing to the medicine inside the canister but to the propellant. Some of these asthma inhalers contain propellants related to freon (though drug manufacturers are gradually phasing out these toxic propellants); large inhalations of freon can trigger a heart attack.

Bronchodilator (airway-opening) inhalers: Albuterol (Proventil, Ventolin), bitolterol (Tornalate), ipratropium (Atrovent), metaproterenol (Alupent, Metaprel), pirbuterol (Maxair), salmeterol (Serevent), terbutaline (Brethaire)

Probable toxicity: Moderate. Ipratropium overdose causes anticholinergic poisoning, a set of symptoms that can make you feel as if you've been wandering across the Kalahari Desert: warm, red skin, dry mouth, and hallucinations. The rest of these drugs cause the heart to race and blood pressure to rise, possibly resulting in a stroke or cardiac arrest. Hyperactivity is a common symptom of an overdose.

Overdose recommendation: No ipecac. Call poison center.

Likely treatment: Observation for four to six hours, with regular checks of heart rate and blood pressure. Emergency intervention with the antidote physostigmine might be necessary for a severe ipratropium overdose.

It's a fact: For a short time in the 1980s, Alupent inhalers were sold over the counter, but they were returned to prescription status after the FDA learned that unmonitored Alupent use in Europe caused severe side effects.

Bronchodilator (airway-opening) tablets and syrups: Albuterol (Proventil, Ventolin), metaproterenol (Metaprel), terbutaline (Brethine, Bricanyl)

Probable toxicity: Moderate. Like the inhalation versions listed first, these are potent drugs with side effects on the heart. Small overdoses—an extra dose, for example—are not a problem. But it doesn't take much more than that to cause side effects. Be especially careful with terbutaline. Even in adults taking this drug, side effects are common.

Overdose recommendation: Call poison center.

Likely treatment: Usually observation in home or hospital for four to six hours. Sometimes ipecac is used. Large overdoses require cleanout of the stomach with a follow-up dose of activated charcoal.

It's a fact: Warning: These drugs are not "cough syrups," though they can relieve coughs by widening the airways. Therefore, only use them as instructed by a physician.

Attention Deficit Disorder Appetite Suppressants

Amphetamines: Benzphetamine (Didrex), dextroamphetamine (Dexedrine), methamphetamine (Desoxyn)

Probable toxicity: High. The fabled "speed" of the streets, amphetamines raise blood pressure and heart rate. In a severe overdose they could lead to a stroke or heart attack.

Overdose recommendation: No ipecac. Call poison center.

Likely treatment: Gastric lavage, activated charcoal, and careful monitoring of heart rate and blood pressure, sometimes for twenty-four hours.

It's a fact: In more innocent days—the late 1950s—the manufacturer of Desoxyn informed doctors that methamphetamine "elevates mood, counteracts sleepiness, increases efficiency, and produces a sense of well-being." Any wonder so many people got hooked?

Nonamphetamines: Diethylpropion (Tenuate), methylphenidate (Ritalin), phendimetrazine (Prelu-2), pemoline (Cylert), phentermine (Adipex-P, Fastin)

Probable toxicity: Moderate to high. Less dangerous than the amphetamines. Methylphenidate is most commonly found in the home as a treatment for Attention Deficit Disorder (ADD), a condition in which children (and some adults) have trouble paying attention in school or at work. An extra dose of methylphenidate—the most common poisoning scenario with this group of drugs—will cause mild hyperactivity and a quickened heart rate. Bigger overdoses can be fatal. Generally, the same is true for the other drugs in this class, though there's far more experience dealing with methylphenidate than with the others.

Overdose recommendation: No ipecac. Call poison center.

Likely treatment: Small overdoses of methylphenidate are usually observed at home. Large overdoses require hospital treatment with gastric lavage and activated charcoal.

It's a fact: Methylphenidate, on the market since 1956, is coming under increased scrutiny as a treatment for ADD, not because the drug doesn't work to increase attention span but because some children taking methylphenidate may not have ADD.

Fenfluramine (Pondimin)

Probable toxicity: High. Fenfluramine is an odd duck of an appetite suppressant. Instead of speeding up the nervous system, it tends to depress it. Thus an overdose can result in a coma.

Overdose recommendation: No ipecac. Call poison center. Seizures can occur within half an hour after an ingestion.

Likely treatment: Cleanout of the stomach and a dose of activated charcoal, plus treatment for seizures.

It's a fact: The latest craze in dieting-by-drug is called Fen/Phen, a regimen consisting of fenfluramine and phentermine. That means more opportunities for children to be exposed to the very dangerous fenfluramine.

Bacterial Infection

Penicillins: Amoxicillin, ampicillin, carbenicillin, cloxacillin, dicloxacillin, oxacillin, penicillin G, penicillin V; also loracarbef (Lorabid)

Probable toxicity: Low. Discovered by Alexander Fleming in 1928, penicillin didn't hit its stride until after World War II. All the penicillins share one characteristic: low toxicity to mammals. In fact, some poison centers don't treat penicillin overdoses, no matter how large. For the most part, penicillin overdoses will not result in serious problems, unless there's an allergy. Diarrhea the next day is the most common complaint.

Overdose recommendation: Call poison center.

Likely treatment: None. On occasion, a poison center may decide that a substantial ingestion merits use of ipecac syrup.

It's a fact: New York's first supply of oral penicillin could be purchased at Macy's.

Cephalosporins: Cefaclor (Ceclor), cefadroxil (Duricef, Ultracef), cefixime (Suprax), cefpodoxime (Vantin), cefprozil (Cefzil), cefuroxime (Ceftin), cephalexin (Keflex)

Probable toxicity: Low. Structurally similar to the penicillins, cephalosporins have the same toxicity profile. That is, they're usually not a problem except for next-day diarrhea.

Overdose recommendation: Call poison center.

Likely treatment: None.

It's a fact: Who said the sewers of Sardinia never yielded anything important to man? They gave us cephalosporins. Giuseppe Brotzu, a public health official looking for an antibiotic to control typhoid, discovered the first cephalosporin in 1945.

Macrolides: Azithromycin (Zithromax), clarithromycin (Biaxin), dirithromycin (Dynabac), erythromycin, and in combination products like Pediazole.

Probable toxicity: Low. While these drugs aren't very toxic, some have harsh side effects on the stomach. Again, some poison centers prefer to treat big overdoses with ipecac syrup.

Overdose recommendation: Call poison center.

Likely treatment: None.

It's a fact: Among Asia's postwar contributions were two antibiotics. Erythromycin, introduced in 1953, was first discovered in a soil sample from the Phillippines. Vancomycin, to this day the last line of defense against antibiotic-resistant organisms, was found in a soil sample from Indonesia.

Tetracyclines: Doxycycline (Vibramycin), minocycline (Minocin), tetracycline (Achromycin)

Probable toxicity: Low. Here's an oddity: While most drugs lose potency as they get old, tetracyclines tend to become more poisonous. Rarely, Fanconi's syndrome, a disorder that mainly affects the kidneys, occurs with out-of-date tetracycline. Otherwise, tetracyclines have low toxicity.

Overdose recommendation: Call poison center. Give a glass of water or juice. Severe heartburn is a characteristic side effect of tetracyclines, even after a small dose. Ice cream or antacids may help soothe an irritated throat.

Likely treatment: None, except for large amounts or for out-of-date product.

It's a fact: Tetracycline was first discovered in 1945. Three years later the first commercially produced tetracycline, Aureomycin, hit the market.

Sulfonamides: Sulfamethoxazole (Gantanol), sulfisoxazole (Gantrisin); sulfamethoxazole with trimethoprim (Bactrim, Septra)

Probable toxicity: Low. Sulfa compounds were originally used as dyes, and researchers figured, if they had an affinity for proteinaceous silk, might they not also be attracted to proteinaceous microorganisms? The sulfonamides fell out of favor once penicillins became widely available, their demise hastened by a famous mass poisoning case in 1933. In the midst of Prohibition, a drug company used a vehicle of diethylene glycol instead of alcohol in a sulfanilamide elixir; 108 died after taking the tainted medication. Sulfa drugs are, however, relatively harmless in an overdose. Trimethoprim, contained in the popular children's antibiotic Bactrim and sold alone as Trimpex, is slightly more poisonous than the sulfa drugs, with mental depression and confusion possible in high doses.

Overdose recommendation: Call poison center. No ipecac with Bactrim or Trimpex ingestions.

Likely treatment: None. It might be helpful to slightly increase fluid intake for four to six hours to help flush the drug through the urinary tract. Some poison centers prefer to use ipecac for large ingestions.

It's a fact: The first sulfa drug, Prontosil, saved the life of President Franklin D. Roosevelt's son, Franklin Jr., in 1936, when he was dying of a streptococcal infection. Another sulfa drug, sulfapyridine, twice saved the life of Winston Churchill during World War II.

Quinolones: Ciprofloxacin (Cipro), enoxacin (Penetrex), lomefloxacin (Maxaquin), norfloxacin (Noroxin), ofloxacin (Floxin)

Probable toxicity: Low. Antibiotics of this newer class, frequently used for urinary tract infections, might cause side effects like drowsiness and headache. But they're generally not a big problem in an overdose.

Overdose recommendation: No ipecac. Call poison center.

Likely treatment: None.

It's a fact: Temefloxacin (Omniflox), another quinolone antibiotic, had one of the shortest runs on the market of any new drug. Introduced in February 1992, it was off the shelves by June after the FDA received numerous reports of severe kidney and blood problems in patients taking the drug.

Metronidazole (Flagyl)

Probable toxicity: Low. Even with a small overdose, it's possible to see nausea and vomiting. But overall, metronidazole isn't a problem. The same goes for the topical gel form of metronidazole known, logically enough, as MetroGel.

Overdose recommendation: No ipecac. Call poison center.

Likely treatment: Usually none.

It's a fact: It's rare, but metronidazole can sensitize a person to alcohol. Allow about three days after a metronidazole ingestion before drinking alcohol.

Isoniazid (INH, Teebaconin)

Probable toxicity: High. Of all the drugs used to treat tuberculosis, INH is the most deadly. Overdoses of INH result in seizures that hit hard and hit fast. Because the seizures are difficult to control, a deadly blood condition known as metabolic acidosis can occur. Fortunately, there is an antidote to INH poisoning: vitamin B6, or pyridoxine.

Overdose recommendation: No ipecac. Call poison center and 911 if necessary. Prepare to go to the hospital.

Likely treatment: The stomach will be pumped out and activated charcoal given. Then, it's lots of pyridoxine. Often, a hospital's biggest problem is mobilizing enough pyridoxine to treat a big overdose, as you must administer as much of the antidote as was taken of the drug.

It's a fact: Before INH and streptomycin came along, a hodgepodge of ineffectual remedies were used for tuberculosis, including, in the nineteenth century, sulfur gas enemas.

Rifampin (Rifadin)

Probable toxicity: Low. You'll get a red scare if you overdose on rifampin; it turns many clear bodily fluids crimson. But in a big overdose you're most likely to see only gastrointestinal problems.

Overdose recommendation: No ipecac. Call poison center.

Likely treatment: Probably none. Large overdoses can be handled using ipecac at home or gastric lavage at the hospital.

It's a fact: Several older tuberculosis drugs remain on the market, but are rarely used. Some may be quite poisonous (cycloserine); others, less so (pyrazinamide).

Furabiotics: Furazolidone (Furoxone), nalidixic acid (NegGram), nitrofurantoin (Macrodantin)

Probable toxicity: Low to high. The least toxic drug in this class is nitrofurantoin. Well-known to upset the stomach, it nonetheless causes little harm in an overdose. Furazolidone, on the market since the early 1950s, is rarely used anymore, although it's effective against a number of food poisoning bugs, including salmonella and shigella. Unfortunately, it affects the lungs, with side effects ranging from pain on inspiration to shortness of breath. The most dangerous of the three is nalidixic acid, which can cause seizures even in small doses.

Overdose recommendation: Call poison center. No ipecac.

Likely treatment: A small meal or glass of fluid will take care of a nitrofurantoin ingestion. It's also possible to treat a small furazolidone ingestion at home, though side effects are unpredictable. Nalidixic acid exposures should be handled in the emergency room.

It's a fact: Numerous foods interact with Furoxone, some dangerously. Any aged product—cheese, wine, vinegar, pickles—can react with the drug and cause severe high blood pressure. Furoxone is also more toxic when taken with alcohol.

Birth Control and Female Hormones

All birth control pills, plus conjugated estrogens (Premarin), DES, estradiol (Estrace), medroxyprogesterone (Provera), megestrol (Megace), tamoxifen (Nolvadex)

Probable toxicity: Low. There's some evidence of long-term toxicity with hormonal products like DES, but nothing of consequence should happen with a single dose, even a large one.

Overdose recommendation: Call poison center.

Likely treatment: Usually none. These products could cause mild nausea, and with young girls breakthrough bleeding is a slight possibility.

It's a fact: Birth control pills themselves are benign—even in a large overdose. But some brands of oral contraceptive contain a small number of iron pills, seven at most, to complete each monthly cycle. While iron pills *are* toxic, birth control packets contain so few of them that there's usually no problem if these are ingested, as iron toxicity is dependent on dose versus weight.

Blood Pressure

ACE inhibitors: Benazepril (Lotensin), captopril (Capoten), enalapril (Vasotec), fosinopril (Monopril), lisinopril (Prinivil, Zestril), moexipril (Univasc), quinapril (Accupril), ramipril (Altace)

Probable toxicity: Low. ACE stands for angiotensin-converting enzyme, a chemical in the body that stimulates production of a substance that causes the blood pressure to rise. While these drugs are extremely effective at controlling blood pressure, they rarely cause a serious problem in an overdose.

Overdose recommendation: Call poison center.

Likely treatment: Unless there's been a large ingestion, patients are usually observed at home for signs of a drop in blood pressure: fatigue, dizziness, weakness.

It's a fact: Capoten, the first of these drugs, was considered so powerful when it was introduced in 1981 that the FDA restricted its use to patients with congestive heart failure. Today, it's one of the most widely used drugs for high blood pressure.

Clonidine (Catapres), guanabenz (Wytensin), guanfacine (Tenex)

Probable toxicity: High. These drugs exhibit side effects much like a narcotic. The strongest of the three is clonidine, with guanfacine close behind. Just a few tablets of any one of these will produce drowsiness or, in the case of clonidine, even a coma.

Overdose recommendation: No ipecac. Call poison center.

Likely treatment: For a freshly ingested tablet, the stomach will be cleaned out and activated charcoal given. If the patient is already drowsy, an injection of naloxone (Narcan) will reverse the effects.

It's a fact: Though it's not a narcotic, clonidine has become a sought-after street drug because of its downerlike effect.

Doxazosin (Cardura), prazosin (Minipress), terazosin (Hytrin)

Probable toxicity: Moderate to high. These drugs have a pronounced side effect: dizziness. In an overdose, you could also experience vomiting and stomach pains.

Overdose recommendation: No ipecac. Call poison center.

Likely treatment: Unless it's a large overdose, careful observation in the emergency room might be all that's necessary.

It's a fact: Hytrin occupies an interesting niche among blood pressure medications: It's commonly used to treat enlarged prostate glands.

Beta blockers: Acebutolol (Sectral), atenolol (Tenormin), betaxolol (Kerlone), bisoprolol (Zebeta), carteolol (Cartrol), metoprolol (Lopressor), nadolol (Corgard), penbutolol (Levatol), pindolol (Visken), propranolol (Inderal), sotalol (Betapace), timolol (Blocadren); mixed alpha/beta blocker: Labetalol (Normodyne, Trandate)

Probable toxicity: High. Beta blockers slow down the heart and cause blood pressure to drop. Propranolol, the first of these drugs, was discovered in 1958.

Overdose recommendation: No ipecac. Vomiting stimulates a nerve directly connected to the heart and could worsen the effects of the beta blocker. Call poison center.

Likely treatment: A cleanout of the stomach, followed by a dose of activated charcoal. Small overdoses caught early may merit release after a short period of observation. Otherwise, plan on an overnight stay.

It's a fact: Scottish doctor Sir James Whyte Black is a modern-day pharmaceutical giant. He not only discovered propranolol but played a role in the discovery of Tagamet as well.

Calcium channel blockers: Amlodipine (Norvasc), bepridil (Vascor), diltiazem (Cardizem, Dilacor XR), felodipine (Plendil), isradipine (DynaCirc), nicardipine (Cardene), nifedipine (Adalat, Procardia), nimodipine (Nimotop), verapamil (Calan, Isoptin)

Probable toxicity: High. Once the darlings of the cardiovascular community, some dosage forms of the calcium channel blockers have recently come under fire as possibly *causing* cardiac problems rather than curing them. While researchers hack out a consensus on their safety, one fact remains true of these drugs: They can be deadly to children, even in small doses.

Overdose recommendation: No ipecac. Call poison center. Make arrangements to go to the hospital.

Likely treatment: The time-release versions of these drugs—more commonly used today—can take several hours to have an effect. Because these tablets tend to be large and extremely hard, instead of washing the stomach out, hospitals will sometimes use whole-gut lavage if a large number of tablets has been ingested. It's a rather messy procedure involving harsh laxatives. The cleanout is followed by doses of activated charcoal and, if necessary, calcium injections.

It's a fact: Here's how calcium channel blockers work: Calcium, a mineral essential for muscle contraction, moves into muscle cells via channels. By blocking these channels, smooth muscles relax, including the muscles that make up blood vessels.

Diuretics: Furosemide (Lasix), hydrochlorothiazide (HydroDIURIL), spironolactone (Aldactone), many others

Probable toxicity: Low. Diuretics increase urination. With less fluid in the body, blood pressure falls.

Overdose recommendation: No ipecac. Call poison center; get some orange juice.

Likely treatment: Small ingestions can be handled at home. As urination starts, replenish fluids. Orange juice is especially good because it contains potassium, a mineral frequently washed out of the body by diuretics. (You can skip the OJ if it's a spironolactone ingestion, however, as that drug "spares" potassium.) Emergency room treatment is not usually necessary unless the patient is an infant, becomes extremely weak, or cannot take fluids by mouth.

It's a fact: Until the late 1950s, the safest, most effective diuretic available was theophylline, which increased urinary output by making the heart pump faster.

Blood Problems

Warfarin (Coumadin)

Probable toxicity: High. Warfarin has its roots in agriculture. Researchers looking for the cause of a bleeding epidemic among cattle in North Dakota and Canada discovered the compound dicumarol in clover. Warfarin, a synthetic form of dicumarol, was named after its patent holder, the Wisconsin Alumni Research Foundation. It's extremely poisonous, but warfarin toxicity takes a few days to appear, so don't panic. Also, overdoses of warfarin are most severe in patients already on the medication, as they're more sensitive to its blood-thinning effect.

Overdose recommendation: Call poison center.

Likely treatment: Usually, a dose of ipecac syrup is given at home, with a possible follow-up visit to the hospital for activated charcoal once the stomach has settled. Also, because Coumadin affects the time it takes for blood to clot, it's important to check the blood one to three days following a Coumadin ingestion. It takes that long for the drug's effect to kick in.

It's a fact: Vitamin K is the antidote for warfarin poisoning. But don't go looking for it in the local pharmacy unless you've got a prescription.

Dipyridamole (Persantine)

Probable toxicity: Low. Children have ingested large numbers of dipyridamole tablets with no evidence of a problem, though dizziness and drowsiness are supposedly possible.

Overdose recommendation: Call poison center.

Likely treatment: None for a small number of tablets; possibly use of ipecac syrup for large amounts.

It's a fact: Dipyridamole does not "thin" the blood. It just makes blood cells less likely to stick together.

Pentoxifylline (Trental)

Probable toxicity: Moderate to high. Here's another xanthine drug, and that spells trouble when it comes to poisoning. As with theophylline, Trental overdoses can result in severe stomach irritation, seizures, and irregular heartbeats.

Overdose recommendation: No ipecac. Call poison center.

Likely treatment: Home observation for small amounts; expect vomiting to occur, even with relatively small ingestions. Full stomach decontamination for larger amounts: gastric lavage, activated charcoal, cardiac monitoring.

It's a fact: Trental, developed for leg cramps, may be beneficial in cancer patients, as it inhibits fever and weight loss. It's also being studied as a treatment for AIDS.

Cancer

Antimetabolites: Mercaptopurine (Purinethol), methotrexate, thioguanine

Probable toxicity: Moderate to high. Cancer drugs kill fast-dividing cells—*all* fast-dividing cells. That includes cells in the intestines, the bone marrow, and atop the head. However, a small accidental overdose of an antimetabolite drug will not usually cause drastic symptoms like stomach cramps, anemia, or hair loss.

Overdose recommendation: Call poison center.

Likely treatment: Small overdoses require no treatment. However, large overdoses of methotrexate can be a problem, and full decontamination—stomach pumping and activated charcoal—may be necessary. The antidote for methotrexate poisoning is leucovorin, a form of folic acid.

It's a fact: Azathioprine (Imuran), a related drug used in severe cases of arthritis, is far less toxic than its anticancer cousins. Even large overdoses of Imuran produce few side effects.

Cytotoxics: Cyclophosphamide (Cytoxan), estramustine (Emcyt), hydroxyurea (Hydrea), lomustine (CeeNU), procarbazine (Matulane)

Probable toxicity: Moderate to high. Again, cellular death is the goal of anticancer therapy. These drugs are somewhat nonselective in their killing, so you wind up with side effects like nausea, vomiting, hair loss, and anemia. Single small overdoses usually don't cause these side effects.

Overdose recommendation: Call poison center.

Likely treatment: None for small ingestions. Full decontamination for large ones.

It's a fact: With Cytoxan, it's important to maintain a high fluid intake, as the drug severely irritates the bladder. Also, an extremely high dose of Cytoxan can irreversibly damage the heart.

Nitrogen mustards: Chlorambucil (Leukeran), melphalan (Alkeran), uracil mustard

---

Probable toxicity: High. Even small doses of chlorambucil can cause seizures in a child.

Overdose recommendation: No ipecac. Call poison center.

Likely treatment: With seizures a possibility, ipecac is risky. More likely, the stomach will be cleaned out and a dose of activated charcoal given.

It's a fact: The nitrogen mustards were derived from poisonous nerve gases used by the Germans during World War I.

Cholesterol

Fluvastatin (Lescol), lovastatin (Mevacor), pravastatin (pravachol), simvastatin (Zocor); cholestyramine (Questran), colestipol (Colestid), gemfibrozil (Lopid), niacin (Nicobid), probucol (Lorelco)

Probable toxicity: Low to moderate. Lovastatin ushered in a new era in cholesterol-lowering medications: safe, effective, and easy to take. Overdoses of lovastatin and related newer agents cause few problems. Among the older agents, only gemfibrozil is a common sight in the medicine cabinet. It, too, is a relatively benign drug with few side effects in an overdose. Not so with Nicobid. Any niacin product—even when given at a normal dose—causes a reaction known as the "niacin flush." The face turns crimson, the skin feels hot, and some people even pass out. It's caused by the sudden release of large amounts of bodily histamine. The flush is usually gone in a few hours and generally requires no treatment.

Overdose recommendation: Call poison center.

Likely treatment: None for small overdoses of new agents and gemfibrozil. Emergency room visit if fainting occurs with Nicobid.

It's a fact: For a short time in the 1980s—and much to the dismay of poison control professionals—a prescription cholesterol-lowering drug came packaged as a candy bar. The Cholybar never really took off, however.

Cough and Cold, Nonnarcotic

Entex LA, Extendryl, Naldecon, and many others with similar formulations; Guaifenesin (Humibid), guaifenesin and theophylline (Quibron), promethazine (Phenergan)

Probable toxicity: Low to moderate. This class of drugs contains one of the few nontoxic prescription medications: It's Humibid, which is nothing more than a big capsule of the expectorant guaifenesin, a drug used to loosen up mucus. Unfortunately, the others aren't as benign. Be especially careful with overdoses of Quibron, which contains highly toxic theophylline. Phenergan, when taken in excess, mainly causes drowsiness, but hallucinations and other strange side effects are possible. Entex LA contains a mild combination of ingredients for adults, but it's too strong a medication for a child.

Overdose recommendation: No ipecac. Call poison center.

Likely treatment: Anything from home observation to a full-blown hospital visit, especially with Quibron. It depends on how much was ingested and how much the child weighs.

It's a fact: One of the oldest "cough and cold" products still found on pharmacy shelves is SSKI—saturated solution of potassium iodide—a drug that loosens up mucus. It's not used much for that anymore, but it's low in toxicity.

Benzonatate (Tessalon)

Probable toxicity: High. Here's an oddball of a drug. Benzonatate controls coughs by anesthetizing the throat. Theoretically, an overdose could numb the throat enough to cause choking. The manufacturer also reports tremors and seizures can occur in an overdose.

Overdose recommendation: No ipecac. Call poison center.

Likely treatment: For one or two capsules, possibly just observation. A large ingestion is best handled in the emergency room, in case of seizures or choking.

It's a fact: Tessalon is the only drug that comes in the dosage form of a perle, a clear globule of gelatin. If the perle is chewed, the medication will squirt out, resulting in more immediate numbing of the mouth and throat than if the perle was swallowed whole.

Dental Problems (see also Toothpaste in chapter 6)

Sodium fluoride rinses and tablets (Luride)

Probable toxicity: High. An aura of safety surrounds fluoride. It's in our water supply, after all. And it's great at preventing tooth decay. But in an overdose it combines with stomach acid to form an even stronger acid, one that can destroy gastrointestinal tissue. Fluoride also depletes calcium in the body, a mineral we need to keep our hearts beating.

Overdose recommendation: Call poison center.

Likely treatment: For small overdoses, a glass of milk will suffice, as calcium binds up fluoride. Antacids are also useful. Large ingestions are a serious matter. After washing out the patient's stomach and giving activated charcoal, blood fluoride and calcium levels will be carefully monitored.

It's a fact: The first two cities to get fluoridated water were Grand Rapids, Michigan, and Newburgh, New York, in 1945.

Chlorhexidine gluconate (Peridex)

Probable toxicity: Low. If Peridex were a stronger solution, we might have some trouble here with tissue damage. But it's extremely weak and shouldn't cause a serious problem if swallowed other than, perhaps, an upset stomach.

Overdose recommendation: No ipecac. Call poison center.

Likely treatment: None. Dilute with a small glass of juice or a soft drink and observe for vomiting.

It's a fact: Peridex, an oral rinse used to treat gingivitis, contains about 12 percent alcohol, as much as some wines. So a substantial ingestion might result in ethanol poisoning in a child.

Depression

Tricyclic antidepressants: Amitriptyline (Elavil), amoxapine (Asendin), clomipramine (Clozaril), desipramine (Norpramin), doxepin (Adapin, Sinequan), imipramine (Tofranil), loxapine (Loxitane), maprotiline (Ludiomil), nortriptyline (Aventyl), protriptyline (Vivactil), trimipramine (Surmontil)

Probable toxicity: High. These are the great killers of the overdose world: drugs that are extremely poisonous and often in the hands of the mentally unstable. Children are sometimes given these drugs as well, especially for bed-wetting and, occasionally, attention deficit disorder. When taken in excess, the tricyclics cause drowsiness, seizures, and fatal arrhythmias, a condition in which the heart beats wildly but pumps little blood. Very small overdoses—say a tablet or two—can *sometimes* be handled at home. But *always* check with your poison center first.

Overdose recommendation: No ipecac. Call poison center. Prepare to go to the hospital.

Likely treatment: For small overdoses, home observation. Hospital treatment includes gastric lavage, activated charcoal, and observation for six to twenty-four hours.

It's a fact: Over the years, antidepressants have found uses outside of treating mental illness. Perhaps the most unusual is doxepin, which has been tested and found effective as a treatment for ulcers.

Newer antidepressants: Bupropion (Wellbutrin), buspirone (BuSpar), nefazodone (Serzone), trazodone (Desyrel)

Probable toxicity: Moderate to high. When it was introduced in 1982, trazodone was all the rage. Here was a drug that relieved depression without causing any side effect but sleepiness. And that's pretty much what you'll find in an overdose, as well. Buspirone came out a few years later and promised to be as effective at relieving anxiety as Valium, *without* causing sleepiness. Neither of these drugs presents a serious problem in a small overdose, although a coma is possible with a large dose of trazodone. Overdoses of bupropion, on the other hand, are well-known to cause seizures. Nefazodone, a new drug structurally similar to trazodone, may also cause sleepiness in an overdose.

Overdose recommendation: No ipecac. Call poison center. Bupropion ingestions are usually handled in a hospital.

Likely treatment: For small amounts of trazodone, buspirone, and probably nefazodone, home observation usually suffices. Larger doses require hospital treatment with gastric lavage, activated charcoal, and overnight observation. All bupropion ingestions are best handled in the hospital.

It's a fact: Food can help block the absorption of bupropion, but eating a meal is no way to treat an overdose.

Newest antidepressants: Fluoxetine (Prozac), fluvoxamine (Luvox), paroxetine (Paxil), sertraline (Zoloft), venlafaxine (Effexor)

Probable toxicity: Low to moderate. Bless the genius who invented Prozac, at least from a poisoning standpoint: It's an effective antidepressant that has minimal toxicity in an overdose. The other drugs chemically similar to Prozac—Paxil and Zoloft—probably share Prozac's safety, but they're too new to evaluate accurately. Venlafaxine may be more problematic, as its structure resembles some of the older antidepressants, and fluvoxamine may cause seizures. But again, these are new drugs and evidence of their toxicity is still trickling in. Many small overdoses of these drugs, especially in the case of Prozac, can be treated at home with simple observation.

Overdose recommendation: No ipecac. Call poison center.

Likely treatment: Home observation with small overdoses. But because many of these drugs are new, some poison centers prefer to empty the stomach using ipecac syrup. *Don't use ipecac unless told to do so.* Large overdoses require gastric lavage and activated charcoal.

It's a fact: There is no evidence Prozac induces homicidal tendencies. However, several murder defendants have claimed that Prozac turned them into killers.

Diabetes Insipidus

Desmopressin (DDAVP)

Probable toxicity: Low. More commonly used for bed-wetting than for diabetes insipidus (a hormonal condition in which there's excessive water loss unrelated to blood sugar levels), DDAVP nasal spray has low toxicity when overdosed nasally and probably no toxicity when swallowed; the drug isn't absorbed through the stomach. However, dizziness and a headache might result from an overdose.

Overdose recommendation: No ipecac. Call poison center.

Likely treatment: Home observation for small overdoses. Large amounts can sometimes produce seizures.

It's a fact: Your second concern—after the well-being of your child—may be an economic one with a DDAVP overdose. It's one of the most expensive drugs on the market.

Diabetes Mellitus

Sulfonylureas: Chlorpropamide (Diabinese), glipizide (Glucotrol), glyburide (DiaBeta, Micronase), tolazamide (Tolinase), tolbutamide (Orinase)

Probable toxicity: High. All these drugs cause a drop in blood glucose levels. Glucose is the sugar that fuels the body's cells. Diabetics have too much glucose in their blood, so it can be brought down without causing harm. But for nondiabetics, a big drop in blood glucose can be deadly. Glipizide and glyburide have an especially long-lasting effect on blood glucose levels, with symptoms sometimes lasting for thirty-six hours or longer. Even one tablet of either drug can cause severe symptoms.

Overdose recommendation: No ipecac. Call poison center. Prepare for an extended hospital stay, as relapses can occur with these drugs days after the poisoning occurred.

Likely treatment: Gastric lavage, activated charcoal, and monitoring of blood glucose levels for twenty-four to thirty-six hours.

It's a fact: The sulfonylureas were discovered during World War II, when a French doctor noticed the sulfonamide he was using to treat typhoid fever lowered blood sugar levels in his patients. This eventually led to the discovery of tolbutamide.

Insulin (all types)

Probable toxicity: Low. Insulin has no toxicity when ingested, as stomach acid destroys it. Accidental needle pricks, if small, can usually be handled at home with observation for weakness and drowsiness. Larger doses need to be observed in the emergency room.

Overdose recommendation: Call poison center.

Likely treatment: None for oral ingestions; home or hospital observation for needle pricks.

It's a fact: Canadian doctor Frederick Banting is credited with the discovery of insulin. He had a childhood friend who died from diabetes.

Diarrhea

Difenoxin with atropine (Motofen); diphenoxylate with atropine (Lomotil)

Probable toxicity: High. Lomotil and Motofen may be the heroes of Montezuma's revenge, but they're no friend to small kids; a few tablets can put a child into a coma. Drowsiness may be delayed up to eight hours, so don't be fooled by an active child who has recently ingested either drug.

Overdose recommendation: No ipecac. Call poison center and get ready to head to the hospital. Usually, 911 transportation is not necessary, unless the patient is already drowsy.

Likely treatment: Twenty-four hour observation will follow stomach cleansing and a dose of activated charcoal. Naloxone (Narcan) can be used to treat a coma.

It's a fact: Lomotil and Motofen have largely supplanted the highly toxic paregoric as a treatment for diarrhea. Paregoric, actually a morphine elixir, has no place in a home with small children. Even small doses of it can kill.

Loperamide (Imodium)

Probable toxicity: Low to moderate. Once a tightly controlled prescription product, loperamide is now available over the counter. At one time, regulatory authorities thought loperamide might cause significant drowsiness. But that doesn't seem to happen, unless a rather large amount is ingested.

Overdose recommendation: No ipecac. Call poison center.

Likely treatment: Some poison centers have limits on how much loperamide is safe, based on a child's weight. So it's possible ipecac syrup or even a visit to the emergency room might be needed. In slight overdoses, however, no treatment is usually necessary.

It's a fact: Don't be lulled by loperamide's apparent safety. The drug can cause death in infants and should *never* be given to children under age two.

The Ear

Antipyrine and benzocaine (Auralgan), hydrocortisone and acetic acid (VōSol, VōSol HC, Domeboro), neomycin/polymyxin B/Hydrocortisone (Cortisporin), triethanolamine (Cerumenex)

Probable toxicity: Low. Ear preparations contain only small amounts of medicine, so you're unlikely to run into a problem when one is ingested.

Overdose recommendation: No ipecac. Call poison center.

Likely treatment: Usually none. Auralgan contains an anti-inflammatory, so it may cause an upset stomach. Give milk, juice, or water. Most accidental ingestions of ear products result in no harm.

It's a fact: Expect vomiting with ingestions of triethanolamine, an ear product technically classified as a soap.

The Eyes

Antibiotics: Ciprofloxacin (Ciloxan), erythromycin (Ilotycin), gentamicin (Garamycin), norfloxacin (Chibroxin), ofloxacin (Ocuflox), polymyxin B and trimethoprim (Polytrim), sulfacetamide (Sodium Sulamyd), Tobramycin (Tobrex)

Probable toxicity: Low. Eye medications contain so little antibiotic there's almost no possibility of a problem unless it's a drug allergy.

Overdose recommendation: Call poison center.

Likely treatment: None.

It's a fact: Remember, drug allergies sometimes don't show up the first time a drug is used. After the first exposure, the body builds up antibodies to the drug; these react the second time the drug is taken.

Anti-inflammatories: Diclofenac (Voltaren), flurbiprofen (Ocufen), ketorolac (Acular)

Probable toxicity: Low. Again, small bottles, small amount of medicine. Not likely to cause any problem.

Overdose recommendation: Call poison center.

Likely treatment: Dilute with a bit of water, milk, or juice.

It's a fact: Stomach cramps might occur with these anti-inflammatories, but probably only if an entire bottle is consumed.

Miotics and mydriatics: Atropine, cyclopentolate (Cyclogyl), dipivefrin (Propine), echothiophate (Phospholine Iodide), epinephrine (Epinal), epinephrine with pilocarpine (E-Pilo, P4E1), epinephrylborate (Epifren, Eppy/N), pilocarpine (Iopto Carpine, Ocusert, Pilocar, Pilopine HS Jelly)

Probable toxicity: Moderate to high—moderate in the sense that a large exposure to an eyedrop is unlikely; highly toxic in the sense that, if one did occur, the results could be a problem. These drugs dilate and constrict muscles in the eye to help control glaucoma, a condition in which there's too much pressure inside the eyeball. When ingested, some of these drugs can cause numerous side effects, including erratic heartbeat, high or low blood pressure, flushing, sweating, and possibly seizures.

Overdose recommendation: No ipecac. Call poison center.

Likely treatment: For small amounts, such as a few drops, probably no treatment. But symptoms of intoxication can be so obscure that any ingestion might best be observed in the emergency room. Larger amounts can be treated with activated charcoal and various antidotes.

It's a fact: Even during the Civil War, doctors recognized the value of a drug found in the soybean plant, physostigmine, in treating glaucoma. Today, physostigmine is not used for glaucoma, as much as for a last-ditch antidote in severe poisonings from several types of drugs, including antidepressants.

Beta blockers for glaucoma: Betaxolol (Betoptic), carteolol (Ocupress), levobunolol (Betagan), metipranolol (Optipranolol), timolol (Timoptic)

Probable toxicity: Moderate to high. As with the oral beta blockers, there's a potential here for significant toxicity. In fact, some glaucoma patients will experience side effects elsewhere in the body just by applying these to the eye.

Overdose recommendation: No ipecac. Call poison center.

Likely treatment: For small amounts, usually none. Larger amounts need treatment in an emergency room, with use of activated charcoal and monitoring of the heart rate and blood pressure.

It's a fact: It might take a significant ingestion of an eyedrop solution to result in a problem. For example, a small bottle of Timoptic contains 12.5 to 25 milligrams of the drug timolol, approximately equal to the typical oral dose of that drug.

Ocular allergy drugs: Cromolyn sodium (Crolom), levocabastine (Livostin), lodoxamide (Alamide)

Probable toxicity: Low to moderate. Almost no possibility of a problem, save for drug allergies and possibly drowsiness or hyperactivity with levocabastine, an antihistamine.

Overdose recommendation: Call poison center.

Likely treatment: None.

It's a fact: Allergy sufferers might remember cromolyn sodium eye drops by its previous brand name, Opticrom.

Carbonic anhydrase inhibitors: Acetazolamide (Diamox), methazolamide (Neptazane)

Probable toxicity: Moderate. When given orally, these drugs reduce pressure in the eye by encouraging the outflow of fluid. They have the same effect in the rest of the body, causing an increase in urination, so they're treated as diuretics.

Overdose recommendation: No ipecac. Call poison center. Get some orange juice.

Likely treatment: For small ingestions, home observation, with fluids—especially orange juice—given to counteract heavy urination. Large ingestions require hospital treatment with gastric lavage and activated charcoal.

It's a fact: Acetazolamide is another of those drugs derived from the sulfonamide antibiotics and is the oldest "modern" treatment for glaucoma, having been introduced in the early 1950s.

Fungal Infections

Oral: Clotrimazole (Mycelex Troches), fluconazole (Diflucan), itraconazole (Sporanox), ketoconazole (Nizoral), nystatin (Mycostatin)

Probable toxicity: Low to moderate. Nystatin, the least toxic of these drugs, is used in small children for thrush. There is little need to worry about an accidental overdose. The same is generally true for clotrimazole. Fluconazole, itraconazole, and ketoconazole are more powerful drugs, but they, too, usually cause no serious problem in an accidental ingestion.

Overdose recommendation: Call poison center.

Likely treatment: Usually none unless there's a large ingestion.

It's a fact: Never combine a "conazole" drug with Seldane (terfenadine) or Hismanal (astemizole), two drugs used for allergies. The combination can be poisonous to the heart.

Topical: Betamethasone with clotrimazole (Lotrisone), ciclopirox (Lorox), clotrimazole (Lotrimin, Mycelex), econazole (Spectazole), ketoconazole (Nizoral), miconazole (Micatin), naftifine (Naftin), nystatin (Mycostatin), oxiconazole (Oxistat), sulconazole (Exelderm), terbinafine (Lamisil)

Probable toxicity: Low. Don't worry about small ingestions of these creams. Very rarely will they result in any side effects, though a large ingestion might cause diarrhea because of the slippery cream or ointment base.

Overdose recommendation. Call poison center.

Likely treatment: None usually needed.

It's a fact: Gentian Violet, an old-time remedy for the oral fungal infection known as thrush, is sometimes prescribed for infants. Parents often panic when they see that Gentian Violet bottles carry a warning that the product is not meant for internal use. However, it's harmless when swabbed inside the mouth.

Gastrointestinal Problems

Intestinal cramps and spasms: Atropine, belladonna, hyoscyamine, and phenobarbital preparations (Bellergal-S, Donnatal, Levsin, Levsinex); also dicyclomine (Bentyl), propantheline (Pro-Banthine)

Probable toxicity: Moderate to high. Poison centers hate getting calls about these drugs, because their side effects are both numerous and unpredictable.

Overdose recommendation: No ipecac. Call poison center.

Likely treatment: Usually observation, with antidotal treatment for large ingestions.

It's a fact: These drugs render the body a desert, so dryness is a good gauge of toxicity. A dry diaper, dry mouth, and warm, flushed skin could indicate a significant overdose.

Reflux: Metoclopramide (Reglan)

Probable toxicity: Moderate. Often given to infants with reflux, metoclopramide overdoses usually do not result in serious problems. Irritability is probably the chief complaint, with some odd muscular contractions also possible.

Overdose recommendation: No ipecac. Call poison center.

Likely treatment: Unless the side effects are severe or the amount ingested large, no treatment other than observation.

It's a fact: Occasionally, Reglan induces an odd and distressing side effect called "oculogyric crisis." Basically, the eyeballs suddenly pull up toward the scalp, so that nothing is visible but the whites of the eyes. That side effect—while not permanent or harmful—usually gets a parent's attention!

Colitis: Mesalamine (Pentasa), olsalazine (Dipentum), sulfasalazine (Azulfidine)

Probable toxicity: Moderate. Colitis, an inflammation inside the bowel, responds to a chemical called 5-ASA. Sulfasalazine, the oldest of these drugs, is metabolized to 5-ASA and a by-product. Olsalazine metabolizes into two molecules of 5-ASA, and mesalamine *is* 5-ASA. You chemists out there will recognize that ASA stands for aspirin (acetylsalicilic acid), and aspirin toxicity is what you might expect from these drugs. And you might get it—except that each of these medications delivers the 5-ASA to the intestines, where it's poorly absorbed.

Overdose recommendation: Call poison center.

Likely treatment: None for small exposures, ipecac for moderate ones, and full stomach decontamination for large overdoses.

It's a fact: Mesalamine enemas are potentially more toxic if swallowed than mesalamine capsules, because mesalamine is more extensively absorbed from the stomach when it's in liquid form.

Gout

Colchicine

Probable toxicity: High. Packaged as tiny granules that resemble cake decorations, colchicine is one of the most dangerous prescription drugs, causing severe gastrointestinal problems and eventually death from kidney and/or liver failure.

Overdose recommendation: Call poison center. Hospital treatment probable.

Likely treatment: Because there's often a lag time of up to twelve hours before vomiting and diarrhea start, it's a good idea to clean out the stomach and follow up with a dose of activated charcoal.

It's a fact: In patients with gout, the development of diarrhea is used as the end-point marker for colchicine therapy. Colchicine is one of the oldest drugs still used; it's been available in pill form since 1900.

Allopurinol (Zyloprim)

Probable toxicity: Low. When allopurinol was first introduced in 1967, its labeling warned that it was "not an innocuous drug." Turns out they were wrong. Even large amounts of allopurinol are unlikely to cause a problem.

Overdose recommendation: Call poison center.

Likely treatment: Probably none.

It's a fact: Thirty years ago, a University of Michigan study linked high personal achievement with gout. Famous gout sufferers include Isaac Newton, Teddy Roosevelt, and Alexander the Great.

Heart Problems

Heartbeat regulators: Disopyramide (Norpace), flecainide (Tambocor), procainamide (Procan), propafenone (Rhythmol), quinidine (Cardioquin, Quinaglute, Quinidex), tocainide (Tonocard)

Probable toxicity: High. Think of these drugs as oral formulations of those injectables usually found on hospital crash carts. These are powerful agents used to stabilize the heart. If your heart doesn't need stabilizing, stay clear of these potent drugs.

Overdose recommendation: No ipecac. Call the poison center. Prepare to go to the hospital.

Likely treatment: Gastric lavage, activated charcoal, and cardiac monitoring—probably overnight.

It's a fact: In an overdose, some of these drugs—propafenone and tocainide, for example—cause seizures as well as cardiac problems.

Heartbeat strengthener: Digoxin (Lanoxin)

Probable toxicity: High. Back in the 1700s, countryfolk in Britain used the foxglove plant as a treatment for "dropsy," or fluid accumulation in the body, often a symptom of congestive heart failure. The foxglove plant relieved dropsy because it contained digitoxin, a powerful drug that strengthens failing hearts. Digoxin, a derivative of digitoxin, is extremely poisonous, but more so in those who have been taking it for some time than in a child who accidentally swallows a tablet or two. That's because the heart becomes more sensitive to the drug the longer it's taken.

Overdose recommendation: No ipecac. Call poison center. Prepare for hospital visit.

Likely treatment: A stomach cleansing followed by a dose of activated charcoal, and, if necessary, use of Digibind, an antidote produced from sheep blood.

It's a fact: Elderly people on digoxin who complain of green or yellow halos around objects don't necessarily need glasses, they need their digoxin levels checked. Seeing these colors is a sign of digoxin toxicity.

Blood vessel dilators: Isosorbide dinitrate (Isordil), isosorbide mononitrate (Ismo), sublingual nitroglycerin (Nitrostat)

Probable toxicity: Low to moderate. Check out the network of blood vessels under your tongue, and you'll understand why a nitroglycerin tablet is absorbed so quickly. But if you swallowed that same tablet whole, little would happen, as nitroglycerin tablets are largely deactivated by acid in the stomach. You could get *some* stomach absorption if an exceedingly large number of sublingual tablets were swallowed, but incidents like that are rare. Isosorbide tablets, on the other hand, come in both sublingual and oral forms, so swallowing them whole could result in side effects like dizziness, headache, and even fainting.

Overdose recommendation: Call poison center. Check mouth for particles of drug if sublingual nitroglycerin was involved.

Likely treatment: For a few sublingual nitroglycerin tablets swallowed whole, no treatment. All other small ingestions can be observed at home. You're looking for signs of blood vessel dilation, most notably a severe headache, dizziness, and flushing. If these symptoms occur, the patient belongs in the emergency room.

Also, with a nitrate product there's always the possibility of developing a poisonous blood condition, methemoglobinemia.

It's a fact: A phenomenon known as the "Monday death" was said to plague the dynamite industry in Europe earlier in this century. Healthy young men working in the nitroglycerin plants had a disturbing tendency to drop dead on Mondays and Tuesdays. To this day, no one is really sure why.

Inflammation

Nonsteroids: Diclofenac (Voltaren), diflunisal (Dolobid), etodolac (Lodine), fenoprofen (Nalfon), flurbiprofen (Ansaid), ibuprofen (Motrin), indomethacin (Indocin), ketoprofen (Orudis), ketorolac (Toradol), nabumetone (Relafen), naproxen (Naprosyn), oxaprozin (Daypro), piroxicam (Feldene), sulindac (Clinoril), tolmetin (Tolectin)

Probable toxicity: Low to moderate. While a few anti-inflammatories turned out to be more toxic on the market than they seemed to be during clinical trials (Oraflex, for example, was removed from the market in the early 1980s after a spate of reports that it was killing people) the nonsteroid anti-inflammatory drugs, or NSAIDs, actually cause few problems in an overdose, with an upset stomach the most frequent complaint. Stomach problems are more common with indomethacin, the old man of the group (on the market since 1965), and piroxicam. But with a tablet or two of the rest of these drugs, there's usually little cause for concern.

Overdose recommendation: Call poison center.

Likely treatment: Home observation with milk, ice cream, or another dairy product to treat an upset stomach. Possible use of ipecac for moderate to large doses. Hospital treatment for extremely large doses and/or when Indocin or Feldene is involved. However, death after an accidental ingestion of one of these products is almost unheard of.

It's a fact: In terms of sales, Motrin was a drug company's dream. So many prescriptions were written for Motrin the year it was introduced, 1974, that its maker ran out of the drug.

Salicylates: Choline and magnesium trisalicylate (Trilisate), salsalate (Disalcid)

Probable toxicity: Moderate. Anything having to do with aspirin spells trouble in an overdose, and these products are no exception. The only thing that saves them from the highly toxic category is the size of the tablets: They're big clunkers, so unless you've got a suicidal person who's determined to depart this life, you're unlikely to see a big overdose.

Overdose recommendation: Call poison center.

Likely treatment: Could range from no treatment for a single tablet, to ipecac for a few, all the way to a full-blown hospital excursion complete with a stomach cleanout and an overnight stay. It all depends on the patient's weight versus how much was ingested.

It's a fact: A 500-milligram salsalate tablet actually contains 530 milligrams of salicylate, the toxic component.

Steroids: Prednisolone, prednisone, cortisone (Cortone Acetate)

Probable toxicity: Low. These products are *cortico* steroids, different from *anabolic* steroids (the locker room–abuse kind). Taking these won't cause hair to grow on a girl's chest or a boy's testicles to shrink. In fact, there's almost never a problem in an acute overdose.

Overdose recommendation: Call poison center.

Likely treatment: None. Some patients may experience an upset stomach. Administer milk or some other soft food.

It's a fact: Corticosteroids were originally derived from a variety of Mexican yam.

Penicillamine (Cuprimine)

Probable toxicity: Low to high. Take one look at penicillamine's side effect profile and you'd think it was the most toxic drug on the market. Yes, it can cause dangerous anemias, kidney damage, and even something called hypogeusia (that's a loss of taste), but in a single acute ingestion it probably won't cause much of anything.

Overdose recommendation: Call poison center.

Likely treatment: Because penicillamine has an unusually high propensity to cause allergic reactions, some poison centers might prefer to remove even one capsule from the stomach. But that may be overkill.

It's a fact: At some point, all penicillins degrade into penicillamine. So those allergic to penicillin might have a serious reaction to penicillamine.

Malaria

Chloroquine (Aralen), hydroxychloroquine (Plaquenil), primaquine

Probable toxicity: High. Deadly is more like it. Primarily used these days for severe cases of arthritis, the antimalarials are just about the most toxic set of drugs you can find in the home. One tablet is enough to cause death in some children, and it happens in a hurry. You've got about thirty minutes following an ingestion in which to get the patient to a hospital.

Overdose recommendation: Call 911. Hospital transport is essential. Cardiac failure and seizures can occur within an hour.

Likely treatment: Gastric lavage, activated charcoal, and vigorous life support attempts.

It's a fact: The manufacturer of Plaquenil, recognizing its extreme toxicity, supplies pharmacists with KEEP OUT OF REACH OF CHILDREN stickers.

Men's Drugs

Male hormones: Fluoxymesterone (Halotestin), methyltestosterone (Android-10, Oreton), oxandrolone (Anavar, Oxandrin), stanozolol (Winstrol), testolactone (Teslac)

Probable toxicity: Low to high. The Drug Enforcement Administration recently clamped down on these locker-room hormones, placing them in the highly restrictive Schedule III drug category, right up there with some narcotics. But these drugs cause few immediate problems; it's the long-term consequences the feds are worried about. So don't worry—a child who accidentally swallows a pill or two isn't going to turn into a "roid" monster overnight.

Overdose recommendation: Call poison center.

Likely treatment: None for an acute small exposure.

It's a fact: Tough tradeoff: Taking anabolic steroids may increase muscle mass, but they can also cause the testicles to shrink.

Yohimbine (Yocon)

Probable toxicity: Moderate. Derived from a species of African tree, yohimbine has gained fame with men as a libido booster. It comes in the unusual dosage strength of 5.4 milligrams, and one tablet is easily enough to cause side effects in both adults and children, most commonly mild dizziness.

Overdose recommendation: No ipecac. Call poison center.

Likely treatment: With mild symptoms, probably observation at home. Hospital observation for severe symptoms.

It's a fact: Yohimbine is chemically related to reserpine, the first "miracle" drug to treat high blood pressure. Reserpine also comes from a plant.

Eulexin (Flutamide)

Probable toxicity: Low to moderate. Eulexin inhibits testosterone from binding to the prostate gland, a helpful effect in prostate cancer. Side effects from an accidental dose might include sleepiness.

Overdose recommendation: No ipecac. Call poison center.

Likely treatment: Probably just observation at home for a small dose, with an emergency room visit for a larger one.

It's a fact: There is little "poisoning" experience with the other major prostate drug, Proscar (finasteride), which is used to treat nonmalignant enlargements of the gland. But it's probably not very poisonous.

Minoxidil solution (Rogaine)

Probable toxicity: Moderate to high. After minoxidil started off as a treatment for blood pressure in the 1970s, researchers noticed the drug produced an interesting (and potentially profitable) side effect: It made people hairy. All sorts of hopes were raised that a minoxidil solution applied to the scalp might reverse male pattern baldness, but for many balding men, Rogaine turned out to be a disappointment. As for its toxicity, minoxidil solution is dangerous. First, it's got an alcohol base. Second, it's packed with minoxidil: A two-ounce bottle of Rogaine contains the equivalent of twelve tablets of Loniten, the oral form of the drug.

Overdose recommendation: No ipecac. Call poison center.

Likely treatment: For a sip of Rogaine solution, probably just observation for weakness, dizziness, or other signs of a drop in blood pressure. Larger amounts must be treated in the emergency room with activated charcoal and blood pressure monitoring. Try to quantify how much of the bottle is gone before calling the poison center.

It's a fact: Cost and the need for a prescription probably helped keep accidental Rogaine ingestions low. But the drug has now gone nonprescription.

Mental Disorders

Manic depression: Lithium carbonate (Eskalith and others)

Probable toxicity: High. It wasn't until the 1940s that a researcher in Australia discovered the calming powers of lithium carbonate on lab animals, but historically there were many clues pointing in that direction. For example, at the turn of the century spring waters containing lithium were touted as cures for nervousness. Today, lithium is prescribed for manic-depressive illness. It is highly toxic in an overdose, but much more so for those who have been taking the drug for some time than for a child, for example, who accidentally swallows one lithium capsule.

Overdose recommendation: Call poison center.

Likely treatment: Sometimes, small amounts of lithium ingestion can go untreated. However, most overdoses wind up in the emergency room. The mainstay of treatment is gastric lavage, followed by careful monitoring of lithium levels. Activated charcoal doesn't bind lithium.

It's a fact: Fifty years ago, lithium was an ingredient in 7-Up soda.

Psychosis and schizophrenia: Chlorpromazine (Thorazine), fluphenazine (Prolixin), haloperidol

(Haldol), mesoridazine (Serentil), perphenazine (Trilafon), thioridazine (Mellaril), thiothixene (Navane), trifluoperazine (Stelazine)

Probable toxicity: Moderate to high. They're not quite as poisonous as tricyclic antidepressants, but in many ways the antipsychotics have similar side effects. They cause drowsiness and possibly seizures, and in some circumstances they affect the heart. Two unusual side effects include sudden, jerky, and involuntary movement of the muscles and an uncontrollably high temperature. Chlorpromazine, mesoridazine, and thioridazine are the weakest drugs in this class; haloperidol is one of the strongest.

Overdose recommendation: No ipecac. Call poison center.

Likely treatment: Sometimes, home observation will suffice. In larger overdoses, hospital treatment is mandatory and will consist of cleaning out the stomach, a dose of activated charcoal, and careful monitoring of body temperature.

It's a fact: Poisonings from the antipsychotics tend to be more severe in those previously exposed to these drugs.

Monoamine oxidase (MAO) inhibitors: Phenelzine (Nardil), selegiline (Eldepryl), tranylcypromine (Parnate)

Probable toxicity: High. These powerful antidepressants have an unusual side effect: They interact with aged foods like cheese, wine, and vinegar to produce what's known in the business as a hypertensive crisis: blood pressure that's gone out of control. These drugs are usually reserved for stubborn cases of mental illness, so they're a (fortunately) rare sight in the home medicine cabinet.

Overdose recommendation: No ipecac. Call poison center. Signs of poisoning may be delayed up to twenty-four hours. Don't be fooled by a lack of symptoms. In a small child, fewer than five tablets can kill.

Likely treatment: Because of the dangerous nature of these drugs, even small overdoses are handled in the hospital with gastric lavage and activated charcoal.

It's a fact: MAO inhibitors were an accidental discovery. Researchers were looking for drugs for tuberculosis and found these drugs for depression instead.

Tremors: Benztropine (Cogentin), trihexyphenidyl (Artane)

Probable toxicity: Moderate to high. Originally used to control the tremors seen in Parkinson's disease, these drugs have found wider use in controlling the tremors caused by antipsychotic drugs—which, being anticholinergics, bring numerous side effects to the table, including dry mouth, blurry vision, tremors, nervousness.

Overdose recommendation: No ipecac. Cogentin has a structural similarity to the antihistamine Benadryl, and drowsiness could occur. Call poison center.

Likely treatment: Could range from observation to full stomach decontamination.

It's a fact: Benztropine has been on the market for forty years, but we *still* haven't figured out how long it stays in the body. So, commonly, overdose cases spend the night in the hospital.

Migraines

Ergotamine (Cafergot, Ergomar, Ergostat), methysergide (Sansert)

Probable toxicity: High. Ergot alkaloids come from a mold. This same mold, usually found on contaminated grain, was responsible for some of the most famous mass poisonings in history. The ergot alkaloids cause intense vasoconstriction, literally choking off the nutrient supply to the extremities. In a worst-case scenario, that could mean the loss to gangrene of a finger or toe.

Overdose recommendation: Call poison center. Hospital visit likely.

Likely treatment: Even small ingestions of ergot alkaloids are treated aggressively with gastric decontamination.

It's a fact: One way to avoid ergot poisoning in nineteenth-century Russia was to look at the color of the bread on the baker's shelf. Reddish bread was baked with ergot-contaminated flour. The redder the bread, the more poisonous the loaf.

Sumatriptan (Imitrex)

Probable toxicity: Moderate to high. It's a bit early to render a decision on sumatriptan's toxicity, but this new drug has been known to cause serious side effects in some who have used it, including heart attacks.

Overdose recommendation: No ipecac. Call poison center.

Likely treatment: Until we know more about sumatriptan's toxicity, most toxicologists will probably elect to play it safe and recommend cleaning out the stomach and giving a dose of activated charcoal, plus monitoring the blood pressure.

It's a fact: What sumatriptan gives with one hand, it can take away with the other. The drug's effectiveness on migraines is related to its ability to constrict blood vessels in the head. But its effect on coronary blood vessels could lead to serious symptoms.

Muscle Spasms

Baclofen (Lioresal), carisoprodol (Soma), chlorzoxazone (Parafon Forte), methocarbamol (Robaxin)

Probable toxicity: High. Sleepiness and even lapsing into a coma are not uncommon consequences with skeletal-muscle relaxants.

Overdose recommendation: No ipecac. Call poison center. Hospital visit possible if a child ingests as little as one of these tablets.

Likely treatment: Gastric lavage and activated charcoal, followed by a period of observation that could last from eight hours to twenty-four, depending on the patient's initial condition.

It's a fact: Until last year, there were no restrictions on the sale of carisoprodol. But the Drug Enforcement Administration (DEA) recently declared carisoprodol a "controlled" substance, meaning its potential for abuse is high. That designation automatically limits the amount of carisoprodol that can be sold to a patient.

Pain

Strong narcotics: Acetaminophen with codeine (Tylenol #2, #3, #4), acetaminophen with hydrocone (Lortab, Lortab Plus, Vicodin, Vicodin ES), acetaminophen with oxycodone (Percocet, Tylox), aspirin with oxycodone (Percodan), hydromorphone (Dilaudid), meperidine (Demerol), methadone (Dolophine), morphine (Astramorph), pentazocine (Talwin-Nx, Talacen); also, narcotic cough syrups: Codeine-based (various), hydrocone-based (Codimal-DH, Hycodan, Hycomine, Tussionex)

Probable toxicity: High. Children tolerate narcotics poorly. Thus, a tablet or two of any of these drugs, or less than half a teaspoonful of a narcotic cough syrup, and you've got a potential medical emergency.

Overdose recommendation: No ipecac. If it just happened, call poison center and be prepared to go to the hospital. If the patient is already drowsy, call 911.

Likely treatment: All these drugs are dangerous to children, but acetaminophen with codeine and pentazocine products are less toxic than the others, and small ingestions of these can sometimes be treated at home. The same goes for codeine-based cough syrups. Otherwise, it's off to the hospital, where treatment consists of cleaning out the stomach, administering activated charcoal, and using naloxone (Narcan) to reverse the drowsiness caused by the narcotic.

It's a fact: Butorphanol (Stadol) is the only prescription painkiller that comes as a nasal spray. It, too, can be highly toxic in an overdose.

Barbiturate Pain Relievers: Acetaminophen with butalbital (Phrenilin, Phrenilin Forte), acetaminophen with butalbital and caffeine (Fioricet), aspirin with butalbital (Axotal), aspirin with butalbital and caffeine (Fiorinal)

Probable toxicity: High. Most often, you'll find these products in the homes of migraine headache sufferers. The barbiturates cause drowsiness and difficulty breathing.

Overdose recommendation: No ipecac. Call the poison center. If patient is already drowsy call 911.

Likely treatment: Home observation is too risky. At the hospital, treatment usually entails pumping out the stomach and administering activated charcoal.

It's a fact: The caffeine in these products is usually of no significance in a poisoning.

Tramadol (Ultram)

Probable toxicity: Moderate to high. Here's a drug that acts like a narcotic in every way but one: It doesn't slow down breathing. Still, it's pretty toxic, with seizures, coma, and cardiac failure possible in a big overdose.

Overdose recommendation: No ipecac. Call poison center and 911 if necessary.

Likely treatment: For small ingestions, home observation is a possibility. Otherwise, it's the stomach-cleaning routine, with the use of naloxone (Narcan) if needed.

It's a fact: Narcan is only partially effective in a tramadol poisoning, because tramadol is not a true narcotic.

Propoxyphene (Darvocet-N100, Darvon)

Probable toxicity: High. Even as late as 1973, it was thought safe to combine propoxyphene with "social drinking." It's not. There are serious problems mixing propoxyphene with alcohol, and in children, propoxyphene taken alone—even a few tablets—can cause death within an hour.

Overdose recommendation: No ipecac. Call poison center. Prepare to go to hospital.

Likely treatment: Gastric lavage, activated charcoal, and careful monitoring.

It's a fact: In use since 1958, propoxyphene has been battered for the last twenty years by consumer groups, who charge it's an unsafe, ineffective drug. However, it remains a popular choice for minor pain.

Parasites

Lindane (Kwell)

Probable toxicity: High. Here's a common poisoning scenario: A parent gets a bottle of Kwell from the pharmacy to treat lice or scabies and, instead of applying it to the skin, gives it to the child like an antibiotic. As little as a teaspoonful of lindane can cause seizures in a child.

Overdose recommendation: No ipecac. No milk or other fatty liquids; these help lindane get absorbed better. Call poison center. Hospital visit probable unless under a teaspoonful has been ingested. Remember that excessive application of lindane to the skin can also result in toxicity.

Likely treatment: Gastric lavage, followed by activated charcoal, and a few hours' observation.

It's a fact: In a rather ignominous honor, lindane, a popular treatment for body lice, was named for T. van der Linden, who discovered it in 1912.

Permethrin (Elimite)

Probable toxicity: Low. A synthetic version of the natural pyrethrins found in chrysanthemum plants, permethrin only causes severe reactions in sensitive individuals. Otherwise, ingestions of permethrin result in mild allergic symptoms, like an itchy throat and wheezing, plus nausea and vomiting.

Overdose recommendation: In a severely sensitive asthmatic, symptoms could be dangerous. No ipecac. Call poison center.

Likely treatment: In most people, none. Hospitalization with life support is sometimes necessary for severely allergic people.

It's a fact: Unlike lindane, permethrin is minimally absorbed through the skin.

Mebendazole (Vermox), thiabendazole (Mintezol)

Probable toxicity: Low. This unusual group of drugs is used to treat such unappetizing disorders as pinworms. Generally, the drugs are low in toxicity.

Overdose recommendation: No ipecac. Call poison center.

Likely treatment: Probably none.

It's a fact: Many veterinary wormers contain the same ingredients as human products. Thus, ingesting a pet remedy is usually of no serious consequence.

Parkinson's Disease

Carbidopa and levodopa (Sinemet), levodopa (Dopar, Larodopa)

Probable toxicity: Low to moderate. The introduction of levodopa revolutionized Parkinson's treatment. However, it was very expensive at first, because it was derived from a natural source: the velvet bean. An upset stomach is the most likely outcome from taking one of these drugs by accident.

Overdose recommendation: Call poison center.

Likely treatment: For a small ingestion, probably none. Larger ingestions are usually treated with gastric lavage and activated charcoal. But these products tend to be mild in an overdose.

It's a fact: Sinemet, introduced in 1975, contains both carbidopa and levodopa. Carbidopa acts as a chemical "cover" for levodopa. While the body is busy destroying the inactive, nontoxic carbidopa, the levodopa has a chance to be absorbed and get into the brain.

Bromocriptine (Parlodel)

Probable toxicity: Low. Sometimes used in new mothers to suppress lactation, bromocriptine is also useful in Parkinson's disease. It tends to be mild in an overdose, with nausea, vomiting, and dizziness possible but unlikely.

Overdose recommendation: No ipecac. Call poison center.

Likely treatment: Probably none.

It's a fact: Is Parlodel dangerous for postpartum women? The drug's manufacturer reports higher than normal rates of high blood pressure, stroke, and heart attacks in women taking the drug after giving birth.

Seizures and Epilepsy

Barbiturates: Mephobarbital (Mebaral), pentobarbital (Nembutal), phenobarbital, primidone (Mysoline); also: Amobarbital (Amytal), butabarbital (Butalbital), secobarbital (Seconal)

Probable toxicity: High. While some patients still rely on phenobarbital to control seizures, the barbiturates—some of the oldest drugs on the planet—are gradually receding into history. And that's good news from a toxicological standpoint. Barbiturates not only sedate the central nervous system, they slow down breathing as well.

Overdose recommendation: No ipecac, as drowsiness could develop. Call poison center. Possible hospital visit with phenobarbital and primidone; most definitely emergency room treatment with any other barbiturate.

Likely treatment: Activated charcoal provides an excellent way to reduce barbiturate levels in the blood, and it may be given several times during the course of a poisoning.

It's a fact: Adolf von Baeyer, a German chemist, isolated barbituric acid in the late 1800s and supposedly named it for his girlfriend at the time, Barbara.

Valproic acid (Depakene, Depakote)

Probable toxicity: Moderate. In the 1970s, the Food and Drug Administration took the unusual step of quickly approving the sale of valproic acid after consumers demanded the drug be made available in the United States. This anticonvulsant had already been used effectively for years in Europe. Overdoses of valproic acid generally result in only drowsiness.

Overdose recommendation: No ipecac. Call poison center. Prepare to go to the hospital.

Likely treatment: Could range from home observation to use of activated charcoal to bind up the drug. In severe overdoses, kidney dialysis can also be used.

It's a fact: Valproic acid inhibits its own metabolism, meaning that over time patients taking it may need to decrease their dose. Otherwise, toxicity could develop even from a "normal" dose.

Phenytoin (Dilantin)

Probable toxicity: Moderate. More than sixty years after its introduction, Dilantin remains unsurpassed as the treatment of choice for seizure disorders. Home poisonings are relatively common, because even with correct dosing of the drug, Dilantin sometimes builds up in the body, causing patients to become extremely lethargic. While massive overdoses of Dilantin are dangerous, these aberrations in blood levels are sometimes managed at home with careful observation.

Overdose recommendation: No ipecac. Call poison center.

Likely treatment: For slightly elevated blood levels, home observation to insure the patient doesn't fall and get hurt. Doses of activated charcoal bring down extremely high blood levels.

It's a fact: Dilantin isn't just useful in seizure disorders, it can also be used to treat some drug overdoses—in particular, antidepressants. Dilantin protects both the nervous system and the heart from the toxic effects of these drugs.

Carbamazepine (Tegretol)

Probable toxicity: Moderate to high. Tegretol poisonings tend to last a long time. Therefore, many overdoses wind up staying overnight in the hospital. Tegretol mainly causes drowsiness. But as its chemical structure is similar to the antidepressant imipramine, it's possible to see effects on the heart as well.

Overdose recommendation: No ipecac. Call poison center.

Likely treatment: Could range from home observation to an extended stay in the hospital, depending on how much has been taken. In the hospital, activated charcoal will be used to bring down blood levels of Tegretol.

It's a fact: Tegretol increases its own metabolism. So, those who have been on the drug for a long time might suffer less from an overdose than a Tegretol newcomer.

The Skin

Steroid creams: Betamethasone dipropionate (Diprolene, Diprosone), betamethasone valerate (Valisone), desoximetasone (Topicort), hydrocortisone, triamcinolone

Probable toxicity: Low. A taste—even a mouthful—of one of these products is nothing to worry about. However, diarrhea can occur with a large ingestion, due to the greasy cream or ointment base.

Overdose recommendation: Call poison center.

Likely treatment: None.

It's a fact: Steroids can be absorbed through the skin. While a one-time application won't result in toxicity, long-term use, especially with large-area applications, could.

Antibacterials: Clindamycin (Cleocin), erythromycin (various preparations), metronidazole (MetroGel), mupirocin (Bactroban)

Probable toxicity: Low. Used to treat conditions from acne to impetigo, topical antibacterials tend to have low toxicity when small amounts are ingested. Be careful with some clindamycin and erythromycin acne washes, though; they may contain alcohol.

Overdose recommendation: Call poison center.

Likely treatment: None.

It's a fact: Clindamycin was once a popular oral antibiotic, used to treat such things as the common cold. However, it fell out of favor after it was found to cause a serious inflammation in the intestines.

Sleeping Pills, (see Anxiety and Sleep)

Thyroid Insufficiency

Levothyroxine (Synthroid), Armour Thyroid

Probable toxicity: Low. Don't worry about a small ingestion of thyroid tablets. Even relatively large overdoses—say, twenty Synthroid 0.1 milligram tablets—will probably result in mild symptoms of fever and hyperactivity.

Overdose recommendation: No ipecac. Call poison center.

Likely treatment: Probably none.

It's a fact: Drugs for overactive thyroid glands may be slightly more toxic than these thyroid replacements but still cause few problems in an overdose. One example of such a drug is propylthiouracil, or PTU.

Ulcers

Histamine blockers: cimetidine (Tagamet), famotidine (Pepcid), nizatadine (Axid), ranitidine (Zantac); also, lansoprazole (Prevacid), misoprostol (Cytotec), omeprazole (Prilosec), sucralfate (Carafate)

Probable toxicity: Low to moderate. These big-selling drugs work well and cause few side effects. In fact, even massive overdoses of histamine blockers rarely cause a problem. The same is generally true for sucralfate and the proton-pump inhibitors lansoprazole and omeprazole. Misoprostol is slightly more toxic. An overdose might cause an increase in heart rate, blood pressure, and temperature.

Overdose recommendation: Call the poison center.

Likely treatment: Usually none. On occasion, a poison center may elect to use ipecac syrup for a big ingestion, or even recommend an emergency room visit. But that would be unusual. Treatment is more likely for misoprostol ingestions than the others.

It's a fact: A study indicated that Tagamet and Zantac can give you a "legally drunk" blood alcohol level even if you've only consumed two drinks. The drugs are thought to inhibit a step in alcohol metabolism.

Viral Infections

AIDS/Herpes: Acyclovir (Zovirax), valacyclovir (Valtrex), zidovudine (Retrovir)

Probable toxicity: Low. Though these drugs have a powerful effect on some pretty nasty viruses, they tend to be mild in an overdose.

Overdose recommendation: No ipecac. Call poison center.

Likely treatment: Probably none, unless there's a large suicidal ingestion.

It's a fact: Despite its low toxicity in an overdose, the FDA recently refused to allow acyclovir to be sold over the counter.

Influenza: Amantadine (Symmetrel)

Probable toxicity: High. Even therapeutic doses of amantadine cause uncomfortable side effects, like blurry vision. In an overdose, things get much worse, with seizures and cardiac arrhythmias possible.

Overdose recommendation: No ipecac. Call poison center.

Likely treatment: Children use amantadine therapeutically, so a small overdose might be treated at home with observation. But it doesn't take very many capsules to edge a child into the toxic range. Treatment at that point includes washing out the stomach and giving a dose of activated charcoal.

It's a fact: Use caution also with rimantadine (Flumadine), a newer drug chemically related to amantadine.

Vomiting

Prochlorperazine (Compazine), promethazine (Phenergan), trimethobenzamide (Tigan)

Probable toxicity: Moderate. Most of the time these drugs are given as suppositories. In an overdose, they cause drowsiness or, depending on the child, hyperactivity. Also, expect to see some odd and distressing side effects, including twitching and jerking of the muscles.

Overdose recommendation: No ipecac. Call poison center.

Likely treatment: Home observation, unless the dose is very large or the child very young.

It's a fact: Got leftover Tigan in the house? Don't use it on a vomiting child unless instructed to do so by a doctor. There may be some association between Tigan and Reye's syndrome, a severe and sometimes fatal liver disease.

Discontinued or Old Drugs

For some reason, people can't seem to part with old prescription medications. So occasionally you'll run into a poisoning problem with a discontinued or rare drug. Remember, many times drugs get pulled from the market because they are found to be potentially harmful, so clean out your medicine cabinet.

For that matter, dispose of all prescription drugs you're no longer using, especially those that have gone out of date. Remember, some drugs—like tetracycline—break down into toxic or irritating substances when they're old, and become ineffective over time. Taking a few capsules of a leftover antibiotic to, say, "knock out" a cold may contribute to the disturbing trend of bacterial resistance that's sweeping hospitals nationwide. Help your fellows: Throw the old leftover penicillin away. For further advice on safe disposal of medications, ask your local pharmacist.

BENDECTIN: For years a popular antinauseant, Bendectin suffered terrible publicity after charges it caused fetal malformations. It was withdrawn from the market in the early 1980s.

BUTAZOLIDIN (phenylbutazone): A pioneer in the treatment of arthritis and gout pain, Butazolidin enjoyed many years of popularity before its discontinuance in 1992. Well known to severely irritate the stomach, Butazolidin was also linked to a fatal form of anemia on long-term use.

CHLOROMYCETIN (chloramphenicol): The first synthetically produced antibiotic is still available in capsule form, but it is rarely used. Once given for the common cold, chloramphenicol was linked to numerous cases of aplastic anemia, a fatal blood disorder.

DBI (phenformin): Phenformin was removed from the market in 1978 after reports it caused severe lactic acidosis, a blood condition related to the breakdown of muscle tissue. A successor product, Metformin (Glucophage) recently debuted. Lactic acidosis is still possible, but to a much lesser degree.

DMSO: Derived from wood pulp, the solvent DMSO enjoyed several boomlets in popularity, first in the early 1960s as an arthritis liniment and then in the late 1970s to relieve joint pain brought on by exercise. DMSO was never approved for these uses, and some studies suggest it can damage the eyes and skin.

ENKAID (encainide): Used to treat irregular heartbeats, Enkaid finally succumbed to a National Heart Institute study that showed it and a related drug might have contributed to heart attack deaths in some patients.

L-tryptophan: This health food store product enjoyed a burst of popularity as a sleep aid in the late 1980s. But more than one thousand reports of blood and muscle problems led to its demise in 1989. In retrospect, it may have been a contaminant and not the L-tryptophan itself that caused the problem.

MERITAL (nomifensine): After being linked to cases of severe anemia, Merital was pulled from pharmacy shelves in 1986 after barely two years on the market.

ORAFLEX (benoxaprofen): This anti-inflammatory was removed from the market in August 1982 after just four months. In Britain, where the drug had been marketed for two years before it was approved in the United States, medical journals linked Oraflex to a deadly liver disease.

PHISOHEX (hexachlorophene): Many babies born in the 1960s took their first bath in the disinfectant hexachlorophene—until it was found to cause brain damage in animals. pHisohex is still available, but you need a prescription to get it.

RESERPINE: As recently as 1978, reserpine products controlled a full third of the antihypertensive drug market in the United States. But a year later, reserpine was linked—later studies suggest erroneously—to cancer in lab animals. You can still get a reserpine prescription filled, but with safer drugs available, it's becoming an increasingly rare sight in the medicine cabinet.

SELACRYN (ticrynafen): Numerous reports of liver damage plagued Selacryn. The diuretic left the market in 1980 after just one year.

SUPROL (suprofen): Shortly after its introduction in 1986, Suprol, a drug used for inflammation, was linked to back pain. It remained in drugstores until 1987.

ZOMAX (zomepirac): Severe allergic reactions led to the demise of the painkiller Zomax. It was removed from the market in 1983.

Illicit Drugs

Obviously, the average home doesn't have a stash of illegal drugs. But teenagers use illicit drugs all the time. Here are a few of the more common ones.

ALCOHOL: One of the more confounding calls poison centers take is from parents worried because a teenager has come home drunk and has passed out. We normally think of getting drunk as a benign activity. For the most part, that's how it turns out. But anyone who passes out from drinking is in danger. You *can* die from too much alcohol. Also, an overdose of alcohol causes vomiting, and a passed-out drunk can choke on his own vomitus. *Anyone who has passed out from alcohol abuse belongs in the emergency room.* Period.

COCAINE: It's been used as a stimulant for hundreds of years—even put into Coca-Cola in the 1800s—but cocaine is a killer that raises the heart rate and blood pressure so high that a stroke or heart attack could occur. Body packers—those who swallow condoms or baggies filled with cocaine for purposes of transport—are especially at risk. If one of those condoms breaks, it's all over.

DORIDEN (Glutethimide): A sedative introduced in 1954, Doriden was supplanted by safer drugs, especially the benzodiazepines like Valium. Doriden produces a deep and prolonged period of sedation that is dangerously enhanced when combined with alcohol or other downer drugs.

GHB (gammahydroxybutyrate): Originally developed as an anesthetic, GHB causes a downerlike effect that usually wears off after a few hours but sometimes includes a short period of coma. Other symptoms include confusion, shakiness, and headache. Weight lifters, take note: Never accept any powdered material touted as a muscle builder if you don't know what it contains. Less than a teaspoonful of GHB powder can result in symptoms.

HEROIN: Developed at the turn of the century as a "safe" alternative to morphine, heroin was thought to be nonaddicting. Just the opposite is true—heroin is one of the most addicting substances on the street. They say it's making a comeback, which will probably mean lots more dead people with needle marks in their arms. Heroin is one of the few illicit drugs for which there's an antidote, naloxone. Untreated, a heroin overdose will kill.

LSD: An LSD "trip" can be a scary sight: The abuser may be agitated, even violent, and will probably be hallucinating. But LSD itself has little toxicity; it's what happens on the trip that's the problem. The most important thing is to keep the abuser calm, preferably in a darkened room under medical supervision. The trip usually ends within twelve hours, but hallucinatory aftershocks can occur weeks later.

MARIJUANA: Look for the laughing, red-eyed eating machine, and you'll find the marijuana abuser. After all these years, no one has a definitive answer as to whether marijuana is harmful over the long term. Over the short term, marijuana intoxication isn't dangerous. But driving a car or operating machinery while under its influence is.

MESCALINE: A hallucinogen derived from the peyote plant, mescaline is used legally by some Native Americans during religious ceremonies. Otherwise, it's illegal.

METHAMPHETAMINE: You know it as speed. It's not quite as unpredictably toxic as cocaine, but speed causes some of the same effects: high blood pressure and a fast heart rate.

QUAALUDE (methaqualone): They've been off the U.S. market for thirteen years, but 'ludes still turn up in other countries under other names and some are illegally transported here. Like Doriden, Quaalude is a downer that can be deadly if mixed with other drugs or alcohol.

ROHYPNOL (flunitrazepam): By now, you've probably heard of "roofie rape." Well, Rohypnol may be the culprit (although some law enforcement officials think it's GHB). Slipped into a drink, Rohypnol induces a helpless sleepiness with a touch of amnesia thrown in. It's not a dangerous drug, per se. But dangerous things seem to happen when you take it.

It's a Fact

- Beware burundaga! When in South America, accept nothing to eat or drink from strangers—it may contain burundaga, a powder derived from a local plant that chemically hypnotizes victims. While on the drug, victims have made ATM withdrawals for strangers and even acted as cocaine couriers. Half the poisonings some hospitals see in Colombia are related to burundaga.
- LSD was first produced by Sandoz in 1943 but reached the height of its popularity on the street in the 1960s. That's just about the time Sandoz pulled out of the LSD biz.

- Cocaine lingo: Freebasing is inhaling the vapors from heated cocaine; a speedball is a heroin and cocaine mixture taken intravenously. It was a speedball that killed comedian John Belushi in 1982. Actor River Phoenix died in 1993 from a multiple drug ingestion that included cocaine and morphine.
- Another name for speed is Black Beauty (biphetamine); Downers are sometimes called Yellow Jackets (Nembutal).
- The first cocaine abusers might've been Bavarian soldiers in the 1800s, who used the drug to keep them alert.

11

Nonprescription Drugs

Just because a drug is sold without a prescription doesn't mean it's automatically safe. In fact, some nonprescription products are highly toxic.

Analgesics

Acetaminophen (Tylenol)

The painkiller acetaminophen is enormously safe. It causes no serious side effects and doesn't interact with other drugs. But in an overdose it can be deadly. As acetaminophen is metabolized, it depletes a protective chemical in the liver called glutathione. You can take some glutathione away without causing harm, but a big dose of acetaminophen can leave the liver vulnerable to poisoning.

Probable toxicity: Not every poison center agrees on what constitutes a toxic dose of acetaminophen. But some poison centers leave untreated acetaminophen ingestions of up to 100 to 139 milligrams (mg) of drug per kilogram (kg) of body weight. A kilogram is equal to 2.2 pounds. So, for example, a ten kilogram child (22 lbs.) can take from 1,000 to 1,390 milligrams of acetaminophen before any treatment is needed. That's about twelve to seventeen eighty-milligram tablets.

"Lots of tablets are gone; I don't know how many he took."

Okay, no problem. First, calm down. Acetaminophen isn't the kind of drug that's going to kill instantly. In fact, in a worst-case ingestion, you have four hours before the drug peaks in the body and another fifteen hours before it starts getting too late to administer the antidote. So take a little time and make a reasoned guess. It could mean the difference between enjoying a leisurely evening at home and a stressful trip to the hospital.

How best to do this? Start with what you have left. This will establish your worst-case scenario. Then, start backtracking. Did you use the acetaminophen this week? Can you remember giving a dose from the bottle? Your goal here is to whittle down the possible overdose to the *true* worst-case scenario versus the panicky one. And remember, the poison center is rooting for you in this situation. They don't want to deal with an acetaminophen poisoning any more than you do. So if you're nervous and need a bit of time, let them know you'll call back with a more precise count. But always, before you give the final count to the poison center, ask yourself whether you can go to bed that night completely comfortable with the information you've provided. After all, it's easier to treat an acetaminophen overdose than it is to treat a failing liver.

Likely treatment: If it looks bad, then what? Poison centers usually have three levels of treatment for acetaminophen: (1) none, (2) ipecac at home, and (3) full hospital treatment. You can be almost guaranteed that if the dose is under 100 milligrams/kilograms, no treatment will be necessary. Ipecac levels are a bit more fuzzy. Some poison centers are comfortable emptying the stomach at a point just beyond 100; others hold out for levels up near 140.

Hospital treatment of acetaminophen poisoning is rather traumatic. Aside from the stomach pumping tube forced down the throat, there's the antidote to contend with. It's called acetylcysteine (Mucomyst), it must be given eighteen times, and it smells and tastes like rotten eggs.

The good news: Caught in time, acetaminophen ingestions are easily and effectively treated.

Aspirin (ASA, Bayer Aspirin, Bufferin, Ecotrin), aspirin and caffeine (Anacin)

These days, children don't take much aspirin because of its association with Reye's syndrome, a sometimes-fatal liver disease that follows bouts with the flu. From a toxicological standpoint, aspirin's fall from grace as a childhood fever reducer is a good thing, because it's highly toxic in an overdose. Aspirin is acidic. Thus, in an overdose, it makes the blood more acidic. The chemistry gets more complicated from there, but we can say that acidic blood affects the function of nearly every organ in the body. Aspirin is also very tough on the stomach and intestines and commonly causes bleeding.

Probable toxicity: Like acetaminophen, aspirin toxicity is based on weight. Again, poison centers vary in deciding how much aspirin is toxic, but you can be absolutely sure that amounts of 150 milligrams/kilograms or greater will be treated, either with ipecac at home or a visit to the hospital for full decontamination. Intravenous sodium bicarbonate helps neutralize the acidic blood in an aspirin overdose, but there is no antidote to aspirin poisoning.

Other Salicylates

To see if a product contains aspirin derivatives, just look for the word "salicylate" on the label. Be especially wary of muscle rubs and liniments like Vicks VapoRub, Ben-Gay, and Flex-All 454. These contain highly potent methyl salicylate.

Methyl salicylate is like a supercharged aspirin. It's about 150 percent more potent than regular aspirin and is thus toxic in a small dose. How small? Well, some of these products contain up to 30 percent methyl salicylate. That works out to 2,100 milligrams of salicylate per teaspoonful, or the equivalent of about six aspirin tablets stacked on a spoon. The minty smell of these products often tempts children to have a taste, and if that's all they take, no problem. But with ointments—especially those packaged in tubes—it's sometimes hard to estimate how much has been ingested. And it doesn't take much more than a taste to cause toxicity. So save yourself a lot of aggravation and keep these products on a high shelf.

Pepto-Bismol contains bismuth subsalicylate, which could be toxic—but it takes a fairly large dose. Ditto for some sunscreens, which contain small amounts of a weak salicylate. (Para-aminobenzoic acid, or PABA, is a more common—and less toxic—ingredient in sunscreens.)

Be careful with wart removers, which sometimes contain high concentrations of salicylic acid. While they have an unappetizing smell and aren't likely to be eaten, a wart remover in the eyes is a painful and potentially dangerous problem. Immediately flush with lukewarm water for fifteen to thirty minutes and consider seeing a doctor if the eyes remain irritated.

Ibuprofen (Advil, Midol, Motrin, Nuprin)

There's a lot of fear out there about ibuprofen, but it's mostly groundless. It takes a lot more ibuprofen to cause a poisoning than aspirin or acetaminophen. Ingestions of up to 200 milligrams/ kilograms generally cause few problems other than an upset stomach.

Other Painkillers

Naproxen (Anaprox, Aleve) and ketoprofen (Orudis KT), drugs similar to ibuprofen, are now available in nonprescription strengths. As with ibuprofen, ingestions of these products are not much of a problem, with food or milk often the only thing needed to treat a possible upset stomach.

Antacids

Two ingredients work wonders for sour stomachs: aluminum hydroxide and magnesium hydroxide. The trouble is, the former

It's a Fact

- Lower doses of acetaminophen can cause toxicity in those with unhealthy livers—heavy drinkers, for example.
- Old aspirin smells like vinegar because it degrades to acetic acid.
- Aspirin was marketed as far back as 1899 and was given to treat joint pain in the hemophilic son of the Russian czar. The joint pain might've disappeared, but the hemophilia got worse, as aspirin inhibits blood clotting.
- Products for menstrual cramping usually contain ibuprofen or another painkiller, plus a mild diuretic.
- Aspirin, naproxen, and ketoprofen have anti-inflammatory properties; acetaminophen does not. So, for example, while acetaminophen will relieve the pain from a bee sting, it will do nothing to stop the swelling.
- Drugs for urinary tract burning and pain usually contain a drug called phenazopyridine, a product normally not a problem in a small overdose (a pill or two). More than that, however, and there's a risk of developing methemoglobinemia, a severe blood disorder.

causes constipation, the latter, diarrhea. Thus many antacids attempt a gastrointestinal balancing act by containing both ingredients. In an overdose of one of these mixtures, don't be surprised if diarrhea predominates. But that's about the extent of what you'll see. Magnesium-aluminum antacid mixtures have low toxicity.

"A whole pack of Tums is gone. I think my two-year-old son ate them." No big deal. Calcium-containing antacids like Tums are virtually nontoxic. It's possible that if said two-year-old feasted on Tums every day, he might develop some problems. But in an acute ingestion, just give a few ounces of a non-dairy drink and call it a day.

It's a Fact

- Antacids *can* be toxic in those rare instances in which the ingestee has kidney disease.
- Milk of magnesia is sometimes used as an antacid. It will loosen the stools at almost any dose.
- Simethicone, a silicone product used for gas, is completely nontoxic, so don't panic if the baby chugs down a bottle of Mylicon drops—nothing will happen.
- Emetrol, a concentrated sugar syrup used to settle nausea, is also nontoxic.

Antiseptics

Hydrogen Peroxide

The safest bacterial-killing solution is, unfortunately, not the most effective disinfectant. Still, hydrogen peroxide fizzes out wounds pretty well and it's better than using nothing. When swallowed, the carbonation stimulates vomiting. That's the extent of hydrogen peroxide's effects. In the eyes, it's the same story: minor irritation that can be treated with a ten- or fifteen-minute eye flush with lukewarm water.

Alcohol

Ethanol or isopropyl, which rubbing alcohol to choose? They're both toxic, but isopropyl is a little worse. It not only causes drowsiness but is hell on the stomach. Fortunately, both types of alcohol taste like liquid fire, so unless you're dealing with a desperate alcoholic (it does happen), a big ingestion is unlikely.

For a small gulp of rubbing alcohol, give a glass of fruit juice or Kool-Aid—something that contains sugar—and observe for sixty minutes. If any sudden drowsiness occurs during that time, go to the emergency room.

It's a well-collected parent who can handle the painful splash of alcohol to a child's eyes. If you're one of those stable souls, treat it at home by rinsing the eyes for fifteen minutes with lukewarm water. Then allow forty-five minutes more to elapse, during which time the eyes should be getting significantly better. If they're still red at the end of that time or the child is complaining, go to the emergency room. Keep in mind that rubbing alcohol won't cause blindness, just irritation. But if you think you *can't* handle doing the eye wash at home, let the emergency room handle it.

It's a Fact

- A speck of Merthiolate or iodine tincture on the tongue isn't likely to cause a problem. But remember that these antiseptics are extremely toxic.
- The toxic ingredient in witch hazel, also known as hamamelis water, is alcohol.
- The hydrogen peroxide you buy in the drugstore—a 3 percent solution—is the only one that should be considered nontoxic. Higher concentrations of peroxide, used in dentistry, for example, can destroy tissue.
- If you have pets in the house, keep a fresh bottle of hydrogen peroxide on hand. It's used to induce vomiting in cats and dogs when they've swallowed something poisonous.
- Once a bottle of hydrogen peroxide is opened, it can rapidly lose its carbonation and thus its effectiveness as a disinfectant. A few ways to keep it fresh include storing it in a dark place (inside a cabinet is fine), screwing the cap on very tightly, and keeping the bottle from excessive heat. As your bottle gets low, buy a new one.
- Betadine contains iodine bound up with something called povidone. The complex, commonly used to disinfect the skin before surgery, is nontoxic if swallowed.

Coughs, Colds, and Allergies

You'd think, by now, that poison centers would've learned to identify those orange, red, and yellow cold and allergy syrups by color. Instead, they rely on ingredients. And that's where calling the poison center can be a chore. You're in a panic. Your child has just swallowed a few gulps of cough medicine, and someone is asking you to spell phenylpropanolamine and pseudoephedrine. The trouble is, these products change. So poison centers dare not rely on color for an identification. Know what's in the bottle before you call, or at least where you can find it on the label. Now, about those ingredients.

Antihistamines

As the name implies, an antihistamine counteracts the effect of histamine, a chemical in the body that causes allergic symptoms: itching, swelling, and redness. Some kids get sleepy from antihistamines, some get hyper. There are even cases in which kids "weird out," becoming incoherent and even hallucinating. But most reactions tend to be minor (except in cases of massive overdose), and many times no treatment is needed. Never automatically give ipecac syrup after an antihistamine ingestion, as there's the potential for drowsiness.

Dextromethorphan

If you drew a molecular picture of the cough suppressant dextromethorphan (DM), you'd find it looks almost exactly like codeine. And that's why some poison centers feel it's imperative to treat big overdoses of dextromethorphan almost as aggressively as an overdose of a narcotic. Like codeine, DM can cause drowsiness, and it responds to the narcotic antidote naloxone. Still, it takes a pretty big amount of DM to cause a problem, so many cases are left untreated.

Guaifenesin (Robitussin plain)

Guaifenesin, not technically a cough syrup but an expectorant—a substance that loosens mucus—is completely nontoxic. But not so the decongestant. If there's one dose-limiting ingredient in combination cough-and-cold syrups it's the decongestant,

It's a Fact

• Among the nonprescription antihistamines, you are most likely to see drowsiness occur with chlorpheniramine (Chlor-Trimeton) and least likely to see it with clemastine (Tavist).

• Some antihistamines are found in motion-sickness pills. Dimenhydrinate, found in Dramamine, was discovered to relieve motion sickness by accident. In 1947, a woman taking the drug for allergies noticed she never got sick on the streetcar while using the drug. Another common motion-sickness antihistamine is meclizine, sold under the trade name of Bonine.

• Guaifenesin, used in cough and cold medicines as an expectorant to loosen mucus, is sometimes recommended for women who are trying to get pregnant, as it thins out mucus in the vagina, making it easier for sperm to reach the egg.

• Spring is the high season for overdoses of phenylpropanolamine, a drug contained in nonprescription diet pills. Phenylpropanolamine suppresses the appetite—to a degree. But overdoses don't accelerate weight loss and can even result in a stroke.

• Many cough and cold drugs also contain acetaminophen.

• It's hard to believe, but as recently as twenty years ago some cold-and-cough syrups contained chloroform as a flavoring agent. Chloroform was banned from use in drug products in 1976 because it caused liver cancer in mice.

the component that unclogs stuffy noses. Both phenylpropanolamine and pseudoephedrine work wonders at clearing the nasal passages, but they also increase heart rate and raise blood pressure. That could be dangerous. So while some cough syrup overdoses are treated at home using ipecac syrup, larger ones get sent to the hospital.

Homeopathic Remedies

When it comes to colds and flu, some parents have cast their lot with the homeopaths, "doctors" who believe small amounts of toxin taken internally will confer resistance to disease. Homeopathic medications generally contain exquisitely tiny amounts of toxins, and this lack of potency makes these products nontoxic, even in an overdose. You'll have to decide on your own whether they work to prevent disease.

Diarrhea Preparations

The safest product you can buy for diarrhea is the kaolin suspension Kaopectate. It's nontoxic. Products made of attapulgite (Diasorb) are also extremely low in toxicity. (For information on loperamide (Imodium A-D) see Diarrhea in chapter 10.)

It's a Fact

- Attapulgite and kaolin are actually clays mined from the earth.
- Georgia leads the world in kaolin production, with entire counties in the state economically dependent on the kaolin industry.

Eye and Nose Drops

"He swallowed just a couple of drops. He'll be okay, right?"

Probably. Poison center legend has it that even a couple of drops of an eye or nose decongestant from the imidazole family (you know them as products that cure redness in the eyes and stuffiness in the nose) can decrease the blood pressure and heart rate and make the child sleepy. That could happen, but it's more likely with larger amounts. The problem is one of unpredictability. Therefore, any child who swallows one of these products belongs in the emergency room for a few hours of observation. The odds are good that if it truly was "just a couple of drops" swallowed, nothing will happen. More than that, and you could be talking about sleepiness all the way to a coma.

Laxatives

Candy and soda for constipation? From a poison center's point of view, few ideas seem as poorly conceived as laxative-laced chocolates, soda, and gum. The chocolate laxative Ex-Lax and the gum Feen-a-Mint contain phenolphthalein: an irritating, rather harsh laxative product that causes abdominal pain and diarrhea in an overdose. But children tolerate a fairly large amount of phenolphthalein before treatment is needed. Some poison centers use 1,000 milligrams as the cutoff point, equivalent to ten or eleven pieces of a laxative gum or chocolate.

Give plenty of fluids as the diarrhea starts. (Pedialyte or a similar electrolyte solution is a good choice.) Your sign to head to the emergency room is excessive weakness.

The soda laxative is magnesium citrate, a product which some say should be enjoyed while sitting on the toilet, it works that fast. That gives you some advantage over phenolphthalein, which takes

It's a Fact

• You'll know you've got an imidazole product if the active ingredient listed on the label ends in "zoline." Some of the more common ones include oxymetazoline, naphazoline, tetrahydrozoline, xylometazoline.

• Neo-Synephrine products contain phenylephrine, a decongestant that causes a rise in blood pressure and heart rate. Observe the same cautions as with the imidazoles.

• Never use ipecac syrup with one of these products unless a poison center instructs you to do so (and they won't).

• Not all eye and nose products are toxic. In fact, anything that's not pharmacologically active, such as lubricants for dry eyes and saline nasal sprays to unclog mucus, are nontoxic.

• Eye rinses that contain boric acid generally cause few problems if swallowed, although large amounts can cause vomiting.

• Drops to loosen ear wax usually contain carbamide peroxide. This chemical is nontoxic but can cause an upset stomach. Dilute with a glass of water or juice and observe for minor vomiting.

• Never give a child adult-strength nose drops. Just a few drops placed in the nose can bring on drowsiness.

a bit of time to kick in. Generally, the treatment is the same as for phenolphthalein intoxication: Give plenty of fluids and observe for excessive weakness.

Other oral laxatives include the very unappetizing cascara sagrada, a liquid that resembles tar; bisacodyl, a harsh little pill (or suppository) that is specially coated to work in the intestines; and senna concentrate. Docusate (Colace)—not technically a laxative but a bowel regulator—works by attracting moisture to the stool. It's nontoxic. Mineral oil, while not toxic to the stomach or intestines, can, if inhaled, cause lipoid pneumonitis, a potentially dangerous inflammation of the lungs. Anyone who develops coughing, fever, or wheezing within six hours of a mineral oil ingestion should report to the emergency room.

Curing constipation from the other end involves such back-door approaches as the use of nontoxic glycerin suppositories, irritating bisacodyl suppositories and commercially packaged phosphate enemas. Ingesting these will cause diarrhea and possibly vomiting, and drinking a phosphate enema solution can wreak havoc on the body's mineral balance. While no treatment is generally needed for suppository ingestions, enema drinkers frequently need emergency-room evaluation.

It's a Fact

• Swallowing a bisacodyl tablet whole will result in loose stools, while chewing one up usually causes vomiting.

• Glycerin is frequently used in baking to add sheen to frostings.

• Do not induce vomiting with a laxative product unless instructed to do so—it only worsens the possible dehydration.

• Rare and dangerous allergic reactions can occur with phenolphthalein. Appearance of a rash is an early sign of trouble.

• Phenolphthalein is sometimes referred to as "yellow phenolphthalein." Oddly, though, it can stain the feces red.

Pediculocides

Nearly all nonprescription cures for lice and crabs contain the same two ingredients: pyrethrins and piperonyl butoxide. Neither is very toxic, although people with asthma and plant allergies should steer clear of pyrethrins because they're derived from plants—the chrysanthemum plant, in fact. For the rest of us, pyrethrins cause minor allergic symptoms: a bit of wheezing, coughing, and an itchy throat and eyes. If swallowed, these products commonly cause immediate but short-lived vomiting.

It's a Fact

• Beware canker-sore products: They often contain high amounts of benzocaine.

• Some cough drops and anesthetic throat lozenges contain benzocaine, but usually in too small a concentration to cause a problem—unless many are eaten.

• Vaginal creams and suppositories used for fungal infections and sold over the counter have minimal toxicity.

• Babies often grab tubes of diaper rash ointment and take a taste. This type of exposure is usually of no consequence.

• Vitamins A and D can be toxic, but ingestions of A and D Ointment cause no trouble.

• Petroleum jelly can cause diarrhea when ingested, but otherwise it's not toxic.

• Ingestion of antibiotic ointments and creams, such as bacitracin, neomycin, and Neosporin, rarely cause a problem.

• Pets are extremely sensitive to pyrethrin pediculocides and can develop seizures with an excessive exposure.

• While it's almost completely benign if ingested, bacitracin that is given intravenously for severe infections is so toxic it's almost never used anymore.

Pep Pills: Caffeine and Ephedrine

Poison centers see plenty of caffeine overdoses, especially around final exam time. Typically, a student will report to the emergency room with an upset stomach, the shakes, and a feeling of impending doom. This, understandably, causes some anxiety, which worsens the symptoms further. But caffeine overdoses are usually not a serious problem unless a massive quantity has been ingested. Otherwise, a few hours' observation and some activated charcoal will do the trick. A tablet or two of caffeine in a child will probably cause side effects, but none serious enough to treat.

Some states are beginning to crack down on ephedrine tablets, sold at truck stops and convenience stores as nonprescription speed. Ephedrine will keep you alert, but it can also dangerously raise blood pressure. Even one tablet of ephedrine in a child might be enough to warrant cardiovascular monitoring in the emergency room.

It's a Fact

- Avoid ipecac with ephedrine overdoses, unless instructed to use it by a poison center. Ephedrine speeds up the heart and raises blood pressure; vomiting can make it worse.
- Caffeine tablets contain up to 200 milligrams of caffeine; a cup of coffee, 100 milligrams a caffeinated soft drink, 60 milligrams
- Teenagers are notorious abusers of ephedrine products, sometimes using them to aid in weight loss.
- The Chinese herbal drug mahuang contains an ephedrine-like compound.

Skin Ointments, Creams, Lotions, and Powders

Got an athlete in the house? If so, you're likely to have on hand an antifungal product, used to treat such conditions as athlete's foot and jock itch. While these drugs are potent killers of locker-room fungi, they're virtually nontoxic. Products include clotrimazole (Mycelex), miconazole (Micatin), and tolnaftate (Tinactin).

Does he have sore muscles? Here's one category of nonprescription drugs you'll want to be especially careful with if there are small children in the house. As mentioned under Aspirin, muscle rubs like Ben-Gay and Flex-All 454 contain methyl salicylate, a highly potent form of aspirin. They also contain camphor, which can cause seizures if ingested. Usually, we're more worried about the salicylate than the low concentration of camphor, but camphor is nevertheless highly poisonous. So is menthol, another popular muscle rub ingredient. But muscle rubs usually contain so little menthol that it's not a factor in a poisoning.

What about acne? Many acne preparations contain benzoyl peroxide, which might cause vomiting if ingested. But as a practical matter, that's unlikely to happen in a typically small, accidental ingestion. Give a glass of juice and observe.

Want nontoxic relief from the itch of poison ivy? Reach for calamine lotion. But beware: There's a difference between calamine and Caladryl. The latter contains Benadryl, which can be toxic if ingested. Steroid creams—hydrocortisone or triamcinolone—are also nontoxic, as is zinc oxide cream.

More toxic are the anesthetics sometimes found in anti-itch and sunburn preparations. Pramoxine is on the low end of the toxicity spectrum, while benzocaine and lidocaine are more dangerous. When ingested, benzocaine causes methemoglobinemia, a blood disorder that cuts the amount of oxygen getting to the cells of the body. Methemoglobinemia hits within an hour, with sleepiness the most noticeable symptom.

Lidocaine is worse: It sensitizes the heart, which can suddenly start beating wildly. That can be fatal.

Small benzocaine ingestions—a taste of an ointment, for example—rarely result in a problem. And while anesthetic skin creams contain only a bit of lidocaine, two straight lidocaine preparations, Xylocaine Viscous (a mouth rinse) and Xylocaine Jelly (a topical gel), are highly dangerous. Even small ingestions of these might necessitate an emergency-room visit.

Pepper Ointment

Its been almost ten years since the first hot pepper ointment hit the market. Since then, capsaicin has become a hot item in over-the-counter pain relievers—literally. Capsaicin is the essence of hot peppers. And while capsaicin is nontoxic, the reaction you see after an ingestion will make you think otherwise. That's because capsaicin produces an intense, burning sensation that's especially severe in the eyes and on mucus membranes.

For accidental ingestions, swish and spit several times using water or milk, then brush the teeth and rinse again. Follow this routine up with something like a Popsicle. If a capsaicin preparation gets into the eyes, rinse them out for up to thirty minutes with lukewarm water. Residual irritation should clear up in another thirty minutes. See a doctor if it doesn't.

Baby Powder

The safest baby powders contain cornstarch; the ones that are less safe, talc. When swallowed or inhaled, talc can get into the lungs and set up an inflammatory process not unlike pneumonia. You can eat gobs of cornstarch, on the other hand, without any problem.

Urine Test Tablets

Keep those tablets diabetics use to test urine for sugar—Clinitest is one brand name—away from children. These tablets are packed with corrosive materials, including sodium hydroxide, sodium carbonate, and copper sulfate. The former two damage tissues in the stomach and throat, while the latter causes severe stomach pain, nausea, and vomiting. *Any ingestion of a diabetes test tablet is an emergency.* Seek medical help.

Those big white glucose tablets, on the other hand, are nontoxic.

Vitamins

"My child ate a bottle of chewable vitamins. What do I do?"

First question: Does it contain iron? Your clue is the word "iron" on the label (obviously!) or anything beginning with "ferrous," such as ferrous sulfate, ferrous gluconate, or ferrous fumarate. These iron salts contain varying amounts of pure iron, the thing we're concerned with in a poisoning.

If the multivitamin does contain iron, we might have a problem, depending on how much iron has been ingested and how much the child weighs. Be as accurate as possible with your numbers and always err on the high side if you're unsure, because iron can kill a child in a matter of hours.

Iron corrodes the stomach so badly that one emergency room doctor described the innards of an iron overdose victim as looking more like razor blades had been swallowed than pills. And iron poisoning can fool a parent by appearing to resolve itself after a few hours of abdominal pain, diarrhea, and vomiting. In reality, the patient's ordeal has just begun. Over the next few days—if the victim

It's a Fact

- To help the fat-soluble vitamins leach out of the body, hold the child's daily multivitamin dose for a time period equivalent to the number of tablets taken. For example, if ten tablets were ingested, hold vitamins for ten days.
- Ferrous fumarate contains the highest percentage of iron, followed by ferrous sulfate and ferrous gluconate.
- Iron is poisonous, but iron oxide—rust—is not.
- Mineral supplements available over the counter are generally low in toxicity.
- Niacin, an ingredient in many vitamin B-complex products, commonly causes a rather disturbing reaction known as the niacin flush: a sudden reddening of the skin, accompanied by warmth and, in extreme cases, even fainting. Generally it's harmless and disappears after a few hours.

lasts that long—the body will go into shock and the liver will be destroyed.

If there's no iron in the multivites, then no problem. The B vitamins, vitamin C, and folic acid are water soluble, meaning they don't accumulate in the body. Take too much and you'll pass vitamin-enriched urine for a few days and perhaps have a minor upset stomach. But that's about it.

Vitamins A, D, and E are fat soluble and *should* be a problem in an overdose, but they almost never are. So for all intents and purposes, ingestion of an iron-free children's multivitamin isn't a problem.

BIBLIOGRAPHY

Anderson, Jean, and Barbara Deskins. *The Nutrition Bible.* New York: William Morrow & Co., 1995.

Banister, Keith, and Andrew Campbell. *Encyclopedia of Aquatic Life.* New York: Facts on File, 1985.

Bendiner, Elmer, and Jessica Bendiner. *Biographical Dictionary of Medicine.* New York: Facts on File, 1990.

Bertsch McGrayne, Sharon. *365 Surprising Scientific Facts, Breakthroughs, and Discoveries.* New York: John Wiley & Sons, 1994.

Borenbaum, May R. *Bugs in the System.* Redding, Mass.: Addison-Wesley Publishing Co. / Helix Books, 1995.

Capula, Massimo. *Simon and Schuster's Guide to Reptiles and Amphibians of the World.* New York: Simon & Schuster, 1989.

Cobb, Cathy, and Harold Goldwhite. *Creations of Fire.* New York: Plenum Press, 1995.

Collier's Encyclopedia, vol. 4. New York: Macmillan Publishing Co., 1992.

Considine, Douglas M. *Van Nostrand's Scientific Encyclopedia,* 8th ed. New York: Van Nostrand Reinhold, 1995.

Dorgan, Charity Anne, ed. *Statistical Record of Health and Medicine.* Detroit: Gale Research, 1995.

Downs, Robert B. *Landmarks in Science: Hippocrates to Carson.* Littleton, Colo.: Libraries Unlimited, 1982.

Dukes, M. N. *Meyler's Side Effects of Drugs.* New York: Elsevier Publishing, 1975.

Bibliography

Elkins, Rita. *The Complete Home Health Advisor.* Pleasant Grove, Utah: Woodland Health Books, 1994.

Ernst, Carl H. *Venomous Reptiles of North America.* Washington, D.C.: Smithsonian Institution Press, 1992.

Feigin, Ralph D., and James D. Cherry. *Textbook of Pediatric Infectious Diseases,* 3d ed. Philadelphia: W. B. Saunders Co., 1992.

Giscard d'Estaing, Valerie-Anne. *The Second World Almanac Book of Inventions.* New York: World Almanac, 1986.

Gosselin, Robert E. *Clinical Toxicology of Commercial Products,* 5th ed. Baltimore: Williams & Wilkins Co., 1984.

Green, Harvey. *Fit for America: Health, Fitness, Sport, and American Society.* New York: Pantheon Books, 1986.

Historical Inventions on File. New York: Facts on File, 1994.

International Wildlife Encyclopedia. New York: Marshall Cavendish Corp., 1970.

Klauber, Laurence M. *Rattlesnakes: Their Habits, Life Histories, and Influence on Mankind.* Berkeley, Calif.: University of California Press, 1982.

Krantz, John C., Jr. *Historical Medical Classics Involving New Drugs.* Baltimore: Williams & Wilkins Co., 1974.

Krugman, Saul, et al. *Infectious Diseases of Children,* 9th ed. St. Louis, Mo.: Mosby Year Book, 1990.

Lampe, Kenneth F., and Mary Ann McCann. *The AMA Handbook of Poisonous and Injurious Plants.* Chicago: American Medical Association, 1985.

Landau, Sidney I. *The International Dictionary of Medicine and Biology.* New York: John Wiley & Sons, 1986.

Lappe, Marc. *Chemical Deception: The Toxic Threat to Health and the Environment.* San Francisco: Sierra Club Books, 1991.

McGraw-Hill Encyclopedia of Science and Technology, vol. 9. New York: McGraw-Hill, 1992.

McGrew, Roderick E. *Encyclopedia of Medical History.* New York: McGraw-Hill, 1985.

Margen, Sheldon, et al. *The Wellness Encyclopedia of Food and Nutrition: How to Buy, Store, and Prepare Every Fresh Food.* New York: Rebus, 1992.

The New Encyclopaedia Britannica, 15th ed., vol. 19. Chicago: Encyclopaedia Britannica, 1991.

PDR Generics. Montvale, N.J.: Medical Economics Co., 1996.

Physician's Desk Reference. Montvale, N.J.: Medical Economics Co., 1950, 1953, 1956, 1960, 1967.

Poisindex (software). Denver, Colo.: Micromedex, 1996.

Preston, Rod, and Ken Preston. *Spiders of the World.* New York: Blandford Press, 1984.

Reader's Digest Editors. *The ABC's of the Human Body.* Pleasantville, N.Y.: Reader's Digest Association, 1987.

Rees, Alan M. *Consumer Health U.S.A.* Phoenix, Ariz.: Oryx, 1995.

Remington's Pharmaceutical Sciences. Easton, Pa.: Mack Publishing Co., 1980.

Salzman, Bernard. *The Handbook of Psychiatric Drugs. New York:* Henry Holt & Co., 1991.

Schlesser, Jerry L., ed. *Drugs Available Abroad.* Detroit: Gale Research, 1991.

Singer, Charles, et al., eds. *A History of Technology, vol. 4: The Industrial Revolution.* Oxford: Clarendon Press, 1958.

Sinnes, A. Cort, and Larry Hodgson. *All About Perennials.* San Ramon, Calif.: Ortho Books, 1992.

Strom, Brian L., ed. *Pharmacoepidemiology.* New York: John Wiley & Sons, 1995.

Sunset Editors. *Western Garden Book.* Menlo Park, Calif.: Sunset Publishing Corp., 1995.

Szczawinski, Adam F., and Nancy J. Turner. *Common Poisonous Plants and Mushrooms of North America,* 2nd ed. Portland, Oreg.: Timber Press, 1991.

Travers, Bridget. *World of Invention.* Detroit: Gale Research, 1994.

Tver, David F. *The Nutrition and Health Encyclopedia.* New York: Van Nostrand Reinhold, 1989.

USAN and the USP Dictionary of Drug Names. Rockville, Md.: U.S. Pharmacopeial Convention, 1990.

Wilson, David. *In Search of Penicillin.* New York: Alfred A. Knopf, 1976.

Winston, Mark L. *Killer Bees: The Africanized Honey Bee in the Americas.* Cambridge, Mass.: Harvard University Press, 1992.

Zenz, Carl. *Occupational Medicine: Principles and Practical Applications,* 2nd ed. St. Louis, Mo.: Mosby Year Book, 1988.

INDEX

Index

Index

Index

Index

Index

Index

Index